Couples
Confronting Cancer

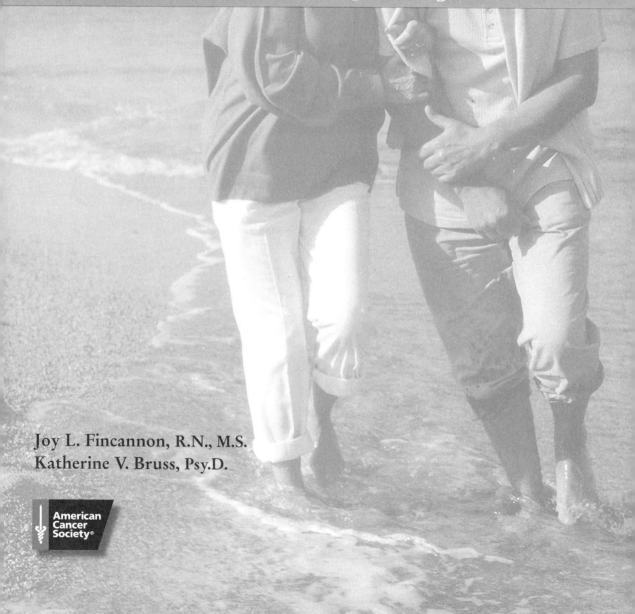

Couples
Confronting Cancer

Keeping Your Relationship *Strong*

Joy L. Fincannon, R.N., M.S.
Katherine V. Bruss, Psy.D.

American Cancer Society®

Published by
American Cancer Society
Health Content Products
1599 Clifton Road NE
Atlanta, Georgia 30329, USA

Printed in the United States of America

5 4 3 2 1   02 03 04 05 06

Cover design by Shock Design, Inc., Atlanta, GA

Managing Editor
Katherine V. Bruss, Psy.D.

Copy Editor
Anneke Smith

Contributors
Lisa Jeannotte, M.A.
Rebecca Jones, Ph.D.
Sarah Feigon, Ph.D.

Editorial Review
Terri Ades, M.S., A.P.R.N.-B.C.,
A.O.C.N.

Editorial and New Media Director
Chuck Westbrook

Director, Publishing Strategy
Diane Scott-Lichter, M.A.

Book Publishing Manager
Candace Magee

Library of Congress Cataloging-in-Publication Data
Couples confronting cancer : keeping your relationship strong.
     p. ; cm.
Includes index.
  ISBN 0-944235-25-5 (alk. paper)
 1. Cancer--Psychological aspects. 2. Cancer--Patients--Family relationships. 3. Couples.
   [DNLM: 1. Neoplasms--psychology--Popular Works. 2. Spouses--psychology--Popular Works.
3. Adaptation, Psychological--Popular Works. 4. Caregivers--psychology--Popular Works. 5. Marriage--psychology--Popular Works. 6. Stress, Psychological--Popular Works. QZ 201 C857 2002] I. American Cancer Society.

RC262 .C645 2002
362.1'96994--dc21

                                                 2002012529

A Note to the Reader

The information contained in this book is not intended as medical advice and should not be relied upon as a substitute for talking with your doctor. This information may not address all possible actions, precautions, side effects, or interactions. All matters regarding your health require the supervision of a medical doctor who is familiar with your medical needs. For more information, contact your American Cancer Society at 800-ACS-2345 (www.cancer.org).

Contents

&c.

INTRODUCTION vii

SECTION 1   SETTING THE STAGE 1
Chapter 1   Cancer's Impact on the Couple: An Overview 3
Chapter 2   The Caregiver's Role...21
Chapter 3   Evaluating Your Relationship 39
Chapter 4   What It Takes to Create a Good Relationship 61

SECTION 2   CHALLENGES..**75**
Chapter 5   Emotions, Relationships, and Cancer 77
Chapter 6   Couples in Conflict...91
Chapter 7   Lifestyle Factors..109

SECTION 3   SOLUTIONS **127**
Chapter 8   Improving Communication 129
Chapter 9   Creating Emotional Intimacy 145
Chapter 10   Strengthening Physical Intimacy 159
Chapter 11   Solutions for Specific Problems 175
Chapter 12   Support Services 195

COUPLES' CORNER WORKBOOK FOR COUPLES **213**

RESOURCE GUIDE 245

INDEX 259

Introduction

❧

All life transitions, such as marriage and taking a new job, lead to changes in relationships as couples adjust to the new life situation. But unlike these welcome occasions, cancer is never a planned event. It is a life transition that is both unwanted and stressful. Like any life transition, the challenge of one partner having cancer can make old problems in a relationship worse, or it can lead to new and better ways of being close.

Every couple's relationship is affected in unique ways by the stress of cancer. The following three stories help to illustrate the differences in each couple's response to cancer. You may relate to all, or only some, of the experiences described in the stories. As you read these vignettes and reflect on your own experiences as a couple, remember that wherever cancer has taken your relationship so far, you can learn new and better ways of coping as a couple.

Three Different Couples Experience Cancer

❧

Alicia and Keith: *Struggling*

Alicia and Keith have been in a state of crisis since Keith's acute leukemia was diagnosed six months ago. He recently returned home after being in the hospital for seven weeks for a bone marrow transplant. They have two children: Elizabeth, age five, and Katherine, age three.

ALICIA AND KEITH WERE HIGH SCHOOL SWEETHEARTS who had married young. Keith always wanted Alicia to be a full-time homemaker, and Alicia readily agreed. But the relationship changed soon after they married. They couldn't help noticing how different their two styles were. Keith tended to be passive at work. Alicia was frustrated by his lack of initiative, and often urged him to seek more money and recognition.

Once the children came, it seemed they were locked in their traditional roles. Keith earned the money, and Alicia took care of the house and kids. Alicia often longed for a different lifestyle. She didn't know exactly what she wanted, but she wanted something more. She wondered whether she should work outside the home. Keith didn't seem to have much fun and hardly talked.

When Keith was first diagnosed with cancer at age twenty-seven, both he and Alicia were stunned. They cried, held each other, and talked about their young family and its uncertain future. Then the intense chemotherapy regimens began. It took two rounds and several hospitalizations to put Keith's cancer into remission and allow him to have a transplant. During that time, Alicia assumed all of the responsibility for their household. She learned how to use the lawnmower and did home repairs she never thought possible. She often brought the children with her to visit Keith during his hospitalizations.

Keith became weaker and weaker with each hospitalization. He put himself down because he couldn't work, and he felt completely demoralized that Alicia had to do everything. Gradually, he stopped working on his computer and playing games with the girls. He watched a lot of TV and slept most of the time. It was much easier just to escape and not think about all the things he was worried about—like not being there for his kids, being unable to work, and all the extra bills and expenses.

As he became less active, Alicia became more active. In fact, she felt like she was running on adrenaline most of the time. She never wasted a second. When the girls played outside, she cooked. When she was at the hospital with Keith, she did the bills. At first, she tried to encourage Keith to be more involved, but now it seems that the effort to "cheerlead" him into activities is too much. Sometimes she fumes inside as she watches him sleep while she runs around doing the endless dirty laundry and cleaning up. She resents it every time he calls her to bring him a drink, but then feels guilty and swallows her anger while she "waits" on him. She has even thought that it would be easier if he just wasn't around. She feels really terrible then, because she knows how sick he is. She wonders whether God would punish her for such horrible thoughts.

Alicia worries about the effect that this whole experience is having on the girls. She has started to give in to their demands more often because she feels badly that they are being cheated by only really having one parent now. She often sleeps only three or four hours per night, trying to get everything done. People offer to help, but she just hates it when other people nose into their business. Anyway, she would rather do it herself, and know that it's been done right. She just doesn't understand why Keith won't try harder—he could at least muster up some light conversation. It seems he never talks to her anymore, and their sex life is nonexistent. She isn't sure how much longer she can go on like this.

∞

Fred and Bonnie: *Persevering*

Fred and Bonnie have been married for thirty-two years. They have three adult children, ages thirty, twenty-eight, and twenty-five. Bonnie was fifty-three years old when she was diagnosed with breast cancer. She had two positive lymph nodes, so her cancer was diagnosed as stage II. Right now, Bonnie has almost completed her radiation therapy. She has also completed her chemotherapy, lost her hair, and gained about ten pounds.

ALTHOUGH BONNIE AND FRED ARE VERY DEVOTED to each other, their marriage has had its ups and downs. Their personalities are quite different. Fred is opinionated and doesn't mind who knows it. His temper is legendary with his children, and he is not always tactful. Even so, Fred makes no secret of his adoration for his wife. He admires her easy way with people and her sense of humor. Friends often remark that he would do anything for Bonnie. Bonnie is equally devoted to Fred, although often exasperated by his stubbornness. She loves his passion for life and his ability to express himself. She is more reserved at times. She has learned over the years that Fred's bark is worse than his bite. Sometimes she just ignores his temper, and waits for the storm to pass; it always does. Bonnie knows Fred is a loving person, but sometimes wishes other people saw this side of him as she does.

When Bonnie was diagnosed with cancer and began treatment, Fred became known as the "pitbull" of the oncology center. He was always her advocate, noisily complaining to staff if, for example, her nausea treatment was not strong enough, or she had to wait too long for treatment. She would cringe at times as Fred was berating the staff for these problems, and then she would quietly apologize to them later, saying, "That's just Fred's way…he's just worried about me. Please don't take it personally. You're doing a great job." She smoothed it over just as she had always done in their social life together. There were times when she became overwhelmed with Fred's intense protectiveness in dealing with her illness. Those were the times when she would go visit one of the kids for a couple of days and just chill out. Despite Fred's frequent calls, she still enjoyed the reprieve and returned ready to be more understanding of Fred and how he copes. As she looks back on these times and the challenges she and Fred have faced and met, she now sees the light at the end of the tunnel for her treatment, and feels optimistic that she and Fred will soon settle in to their normal lives.

⚭

Yvonne and Bob: *Growing*

Yvonne and Bob met eight years ago. They married after a year of close friendship. Each had been divorced for several years. They often enjoy visiting their four children from their previous marriage. Four months ago, Bob was diagnosed with lung cancer. He recently received the startling news that the cancer has spread to his liver. He is undergoing chemotherapy, but he and Yvonne both know that it is likely he will not recover. He is weak, feels sick, and has lost about thirty pounds.

WHEN YVONNE AND BOB FIRST MET, they quickly discovered they were kindred spirits, having been through unsuccessful relationships. Now in their sixties, they have spent the past seven years enjoying Bob's early retirement. They traveled the world, wined and dined, and hiked many trails. The companionship that they share is very peaceful and rarely disturbed by complicated discussions or arguments. Because he and Yvonne must stay close to home now, they rarely get out to do the things that they used to enjoy. So it is surprising that today they sometimes joke, "Hey, cancer is the best thing that ever happened to us!"

Bob went through moments of intense sadness after his diagnosis and at first felt very angry about having the cancer. He even questioned his religious faith at times; getting cancer felt so unfair. Having now come out the other side of these painful feelings, Bob might say that his diagnosis was ultimately a "wake-up call" that led him to question the meaning of his life and of this whole experience, even to wonder about spiritual issues he didn't usually think about.

Most importantly, he turned to Yvonne to explore these issues with him, for example, reading or praying together or discussing the meaning of it all. They began to incorporate time into their daily schedules to reflect together. No matter what was happening, they read, prayed, or just were silent together at these times. They found a deeper connection by sharing reflections about meaningful issues, not just everyday matters. They began talking about all the important things they had never brought up: their disappointments, childhood memories, and deepest fears. Their love became stronger and richer as they shared these discussions. They both remarked that they had never known a relationship could be so satisfying and close; neither had ever experienced it. Even though they were going through this terrible cancer experience, they still had each other. And as a couple, they were thriving.

Soon after Bob's diagnosis, they met another couple, Ted and Ann, who had been through a similar journey with Ann's cancer. They began spending time with them, eating at each other's houses, playing cards, and actually laughing openly about some of the experiences that come with the process of having cancer and treatment. Having dealt with cancer themselves, Ted and Ann understood that it was okay to talk and laugh about the cancer, so Bob and Yvonne felt they could be themselves—happy, sad, frustrated, or giddy. Ted and Ann understood all of these feelings.

Since Bob had to be hospitalized a couple of times, the four grown kids from their two different families, who had always gone their separate ways, were forced to spend more time together. When the children saw how close Bob and Yvonne had become, they shared their amazement and delight with one another. Although the children were painfully grieved by Bob's illness, they were comforted to know that he and Yvonne had found strength in each other and their shared reflections on the experience. Knowing that cancer had prompted Bob and Yvonne to explore the deeper meaning in the experience evoked similar contemplation in their own lives, and even led to closer relationships among them.

Every Couple Is Different

For Bob and Yvonne, the process of going through such pain and grief and coping with it together actually prompted a kind of growth, leading their relationships with each other and with others in their lives to become closer. Instead of staying the same, like Fred and Bonnie (which was a success in its own way), or falling apart (as with Alicia and Keith), Yvonne and Bob actually grew through the cancer experience by turning to each other to find meaning in the experience.

Don't worry if you can't relate to Yvonne and Bob's experience right now. The stress of cancer affects all relationships differently. Still, there may be something to be learned from what Bob and Yvonne did that helped strengthen their relationship in the face of a challenge. The ways they improved their relationship, and other important strategies, are covered in this book. Even if your relationship is having ups and downs, this book will help you to improve your communication and cope better with the difficult times.

Marriage Is Tough

Most of us have heard the discouraging statistics on marriage. One in two marriages in the United States ends in divorce. Each year, two million adults and one million children in this country are affected by divorce. Couples increasingly view staying married as a voluntary decision, and the stigma of divorce has diminished.

Roles within the family are also changing. For example, women are now better able to provide for themselves financially and to raise a family without a partner, and men are more often primary caretakers for their children. Couples have had to adapt to these changes. When the stresses of life—such as juggling kids and careers—become overwhelming, partners may ignore the quality of their relationship. While the reasons for the changing family structure in our society are complicated and we can't do justice to them here, the bottom line is this: maintaining a committed intimate relationship is not easy!

When Cancer Enters the Picture

Along comes cancer to stir things up even further. By all accounts, cancer is a life-changing experience—one that no one plans. As you can see from our three couples' stories, the experience of cancer can be life affirming or destructive (or, at times, both). But minimally, it is a sobering—not to mention time-consuming—experience, and often a source of seemingly unrelenting stress on a family.

Cancer can be frightening not only to the person who is diagnosed, but also to the spouse or partner. Couples often strive to make their relationship work even in the best of times. When cancer enters the picture, relationships can become even more strained. This book was written to help couples cope with the stress placed on relationships when a spouse or partner has been diagnosed with cancer, and to help couples deal with cancer more successfully. What you will find in this book are practical methods you can use to improve your relationship, both during and beyond the cancer experience.

In this book, we provide information about how many couples experience cancer: the problems it often causes, how to solve those problems, even how to prevent them. We offer methods throughout the book that may help you become closer to your partner, communicating more easily and openly with one another. Here's an overview of the important topics that are covered in this book.

How This Book Is Organized

&c.

Section 1: *Setting the Stage*

In the first chapter, we explain what the person with cancer is going through, as well as how cancer impacts couples' relationships—married or not. You'll see how particular types of cancer may present unique issues for couples. We also explore how culture and family backgrounds influence coping styles in couples who are dealing with cancer.

In Chapter 2, we address the partner who doesn't have cancer, the person in the caregiver role. What are the caregiver's feelings and needs? What might he or she experience while watching a loved one go through a life-threatening illness?

In Chapter 3, we take you through the process of evaluating your own relationship. How do you communicate as a couple? How committed are you to each other? What are the sexual and intimate aspects of your relationship like? How dependent on each other do you feel? What are your individual approaches to raising children and how do they impact your relationship? How does being male or female affect your interaction?

Because it is important to understand what a good or satisfying relationship is, we share the latest research about what it takes to make a good relationship in Chapter 4. We describe the life stages of a typical relationship. In this chapter, we focus on the positive side of relationships—the strengths that relationships can offer in a crisis, and a description of what it is like to deal *effectively* with a crisis. We also provide an understanding of how each partner's family background may influence a couple's relationship.

୫ଓ

Section 2: *Challenges*

There are many challenges to face when dealing with cancer. Emotional reactions to cancer can lead to problems with intimacy or magnify problems you already have, which we discuss in Chapter 5. Depression and anxiety may occur or worsen in the person diagnosed with cancer or their significant other, affecting the individual as well as the couple. Anger and power struggles in couples may develop or grow worse through the stress of treatment and its aftermath.

Sometimes, one partner complains that the other seems "emotionally unavailable" or distant; the person viewed as distant may be either the partner with cancer or the partner without cancer, for different reasons. Over time, this emotional distance can be damaging to the relationship if it is not addressed. Sexual problems and changes are common in couples with cancer and may occur as a result of the difficulties with emotional closeness while coping with cancer, as well as the result of direct physical effects of cancer and its medical treatment. We discuss all of these problems in this chapter in detail.

Chapter 6 deals with couples who feel "stuck" or unable to move forward either together or apart. Some couples may be dealing with infidelity, drug or alcohol problems, domestic violence, or even divorce. Such problems may be separate from the experience of having cancer, but they often can add a great deal of stress to a cancer patient's life.

A variety of lifestyle concerns are addressed in Chapter 7. Here we explore couples' concerns about parenting. Stepfamilies and blended families are very common, and they have unique issues, which we discuss. For more information on this topic, you can read *Cancer in the Family: Helping Children Cope with a Parent's Illness* (see the *Resource Guide* at the end of this book). We also address the particular challenges faced by dual-career and same-sex couples. With this chapter we begin to transition from focusing on all of the challenges couples must face to focusing on ways to manage them.

۳۴

Section 3: *Solutions*

You may find yourself beginning to feel overwhelmed by the problems described in Section 2. In Section 3, however, we offer some practical methods to help you cope with these problems and strengthen your relationship. The stress of dealing with cancer can hinder communication skills, even in couples who are used to being open with one another. In Chapter 8, we explain how to create more closeness in a relationship and strengthen communication. We also offer suggestions for ways to reach compromises and resolve conflicts.

Once the groundwork of solid communication is set, couples can begin to develop more intimacy and closeness. In Chapter 9, we explore ways couples can find common ground to create more emotional intimacy. Couples can reach deeper levels in their relationship by learning how to be more open and direct. Part of the process involves being completely honest about how each partner feels about having to face cancer. The role of spirituality in relationships is also highlighted.

Physical intimacy is the focus of Chapter 10. Couples often worry about how their sexual relationship will be affected by cancer. We discuss how couples can overcome anxiety about sex during and after cancer treatment. This chapter also explores ways to keep your sexual relationship strong during and after cancer treatment.

In Chapter 11, we discuss solutions related to specific issues raised earlier, such as infertility, infidelity, domestic violence, alcohol and drug issues, and divorce. We also offer some suggestions for dual-career and same-sex couples who are facing cancer.

Chapter 12 explains the support services that are available to couples—ranging from couples therapy to support groups. Here we provide guidelines for when to seek help and outline the signs to look for when a relationship is in trouble. The *Resource Guide* at the end of the book directs couples to additional sources for information and support.

Couples' Corner is a special workbook filled with exercises couples can use to work through their experiences within the framework of an intimate relationship. Some of the exercises are designed to be completed individually, while others are meant to be done together.

∞

Congratulations on starting this book! It is not always easy to think about relationship problems, especially in the middle of a cancer crisis. But you have taken the first step to actually growing through the cancer experience as a couple—rather than merely surviving it.

SECTION 1
Setting the Stage

In this section, we provide the backdrop for understanding how you and your partner relate to each other as a couple. When you are dealing with cancer, it is even more important to understand how you can work together to get through the challenges of a serious disease.

Here we explore the impact of cancer, the caregiver's role, and the key ingredients of a good relationship, which can carry you through treatment and beyond. We also offer some suggestions for evaluating your own relationship. You'll be able to identify problem areas you or your partner may have in establishing or maintaining good communication. We'll also help you to identify strengths in your relationship, and we'll suggest strategies for building on these strengths.

Chapter One

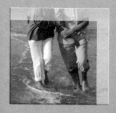

Cancer's Impact
on the Couple: An Overview

The stories in the Introduction show the dramatic effect that cancer can have on couples. In this chapter, we'll look at more specific details about how cancer affects both people within a relationship, as well as how different coping styles and cultural backgrounds can affect relationships during stressful times. We explore the psychological impact of cancer by looking at what we know through our experience working with couples, and through research findings. Many of these findings have come from the growing field of "psycho-oncology," or the psychology of cancer.

How Both People Are Affected
Throughout the Process

As you undoubtedly realize by now, cancer happens to the couple, not just to the individual. While you and your partner will each react to and cope with the experience of cancer in unique ways, both of you will be affected by it.

Diagnosis

Patients and their partners often react to the diagnosis of cancer with feelings of shock and disappointment, even betrayal. Each member of the couple adjusts priorities to make room for the new, unwanted reality of cancer and its treatment.

Naturally, your reaction to the diagnosis will depend upon the specific medical information you are given. You may feel like you are on an emotional roller coaster as information is revealed concerning the type of cancer, its stage of progression, and the likelihood of a good response to treatment. No matter how hopeful the outlook, it is natural for you and your partner to have fears about what cancer will bring. Despite medical advances in the treatment of cancer, people diagnosed with cancer are forced to consider the possibility of long-term illness, death, and other effects of cancer. One psychiatrist who works with cancer patients, Lynna Lesko, M.D., Ph.D., has described the most common fears as "the six Ds:"

- Death
- Dependence
- Disfigurement
- Disruption
- Disability
- Discomfort

At this point in the process, you probably have strong feelings about the impact cancer may have on both yourself and your partner. Patients typically feel badly for themselves as well as for their partners who are forced to go through this. Healthy partners or spouses feel sad that their loved ones will be going through such a tough experience, and also may feel bereft at the thought of possibly losing their partner and certainly enduring a major disruption in their once peaceful shared life as a couple.

Following on the heels of those feelings are waves of guilt about having "selfish" thoughts that are often experienced by both patients and their partners. The healthy partner—or even the patient—may feel it is wrong to have self-focused concerns. Both partners may blame themselves for the cancer, thinking, "I should have taken better care of myself" or—on the other side of the coin—"I should have taken better care of my partner." It's hard to say which is more difficult—blaming yourself or feeling helpless. Both can be tough and painful.

In addition to the diagnosis and the anxiety it brings, there are a lot of other unwanted hurdles. Both partners may worry about how to tell other family members or children. Immediately following the diagnosis, couples must think about their financial and work situations and how to manage the crisis. Either partner may simply feel angry about having to go through cancer (we'll talk more about dealing with anger in Chapter 5).

After the diagnosis, there are a lot of decisions to be made. Who will offer a second opinion or treat the person diagnosed with cancer? What type of treatment should he or she receive? How will we handle the treatment schedule? Do we need genetic counseling if genetic inheritance for the disease is suspected? Are there any complementary treatments to consider? It can seem nearly impossible to make all of these decisions calmly and cooperatively as a couple just when you are feeling on edge from the stress of the diagnosis.

Treatment

During the treatment phase, the particular challenges you will face depend on the specific treatment process, its length, and anticipated side effects. Few side effects impact couples more than fatigue, which is one of the most common side effects of cancer treatment. Every aspect of a couple's life is affected by how much energy the person with cancer has to cope with household tasks. If the person with cancer has minimal energy, the healthy partner will need to pick up the slack. When the healthy partner is doing more to help out at home, there can be a "ripple effect" throughout the family and even with coworkers at the office, as older children and coworkers may scramble to relieve some of the burden for the healthy partner. In the first couple described in the Introduction, Alicia picked up all the slack for Keith, who was both depressed and physically less able to do daily household maintenance. As a result, Alicia felt frustrated, angry, and guilty.

Just as in the diagnosis phase, the treatment phase may bring many ups and downs, and even small crises. These include things like an unexpected hospitalization, an unusual and troublesome side effect of treatment, or an unexpected finding on a scan. Each hurdle requires cooperative problem solving and mutual support between you and your partner.

These stresses often challenge even a strong relationship. Fred and Bonnie (the second couple described in the Introduction) had several of these "bumps in the road" to contend with throughout Bonnie's treatment. Unlike younger couples, Fred and Bonnie had more than thirty years of experience dealing with life's "curve balls" together before Bonnie's diagnosis with cancer. So when Fred got terribly upset and nervous in the face of an unexpected hospitalization, Bonnie knew from years of experience how to deal with his distress. She allowed him to express his feelings, and then (when the timing was right) would gently ask him to try to relax. This worked for them as it had so many times before.

What works for you and your partner will depend on your personalities and how each of you tends to cope with stress and strong feelings. It is probably helpful to assume that you and your partner differ in your preferred ways of coping. One of you may express feelings loudly, while the other may be silent or withdrawn. We will talk more about understanding differences in coping later in this chapter. Specifically, we will talk about how your coping styles may be influenced by role changes, as well as by your ethnic and family background, and how the differences in your backgrounds may impact your efforts to understand and support each other.

After Treatment

Even after treatment, cancer does not vanish from couples' lives. Often, the world feels less predictable after the unsettling experience of cancer, and there is the threat of a relapse or recurrence. Some people respond to this threat by making more time for each other and for other family members. Although making time to be close is a positive way to cope, it is also natural not to feel altogether positive about having experienced cancer. Some people who have had cancer and their partners feel consumed with fear that lightning will strike twice. Couples sometimes have a hard time feeling comfortable planning for a long-term future.

Still, other couples are ultimately able to come out the other side of the fear and anger, and their relationships can actually grow through the struggle. This was the case for Yvonne and Bob (the third couple in the Introduction), who were able to move beyond their experience with cancer. Even though the outcome was not very hopeful, both partners were able to evaluate themselves and find more meaning in their lives. Sharing that meaning was very special to them both. For example, Yvonne always had a concrete and practical approach to life. But with Bob's cancer, she realized there were many events beyond her control. She began to feel the presence of something inside her that gave her strength and support. She sensed that this came from somewhere else and was not just her own inner reserves. With that realization and further spiritual exploration, Yvonne found a coping skill that served her well in other areas of her life.

The Healthy Partner or Caregiver

What does the healthy partner or caregiver feel when a loved one has cancer? What does he or she think about? In research studies, spouses of people with cancer have reported feelings of loss of control, uncertainty, and helplessness. In group therapy, the partners of people with cancer tend to bring up certain issues again and again. These recurring themes include:

- Providing physical care
- Dealing with fear, emotional pain, loneliness, and suffering
- Feelings of inadequacy as the caregiver
- Difficulty with showing emotions or being close
- Different cultural and religious practices
- Having young children who need attention
- Personal family issues or family history
- Guilt about having good health
- Resentment of the ill partner's demands
- Boredom with a long illness or treatment process
- Facing death
- How to say goodbye to each other and family members

Overall, the stresses involved in caregiving are similar for men and women. Research suggests that for both genders, the caregiver (the spouse or partner who is not ill) may actually feel more upset about the cancer than the partner who is ill with cancer. For example, studies of breast cancer's effect on couples suggest that a breast cancer diagnosis may be just as upsetting to the partner as it is to the patient.

Some studies suggest there may be some gender differences in the experiences of caregivers. For example, one study found that wives actually coped better with having a terminal illness than their husbands. Another study reported that men who were caregivers derived more satisfaction from the experience of caring for a spouse than did female caregivers. There is also some evidence from research that men may be more likely than women to withdraw from others when a spouse is diagnosed with cancer, and may be less comfortable receiving help from others.

However, we should not jump to making generalizations or stereotypes based on a small number of research studies. A false stereotype about men is that they need less support than women, or that men are stoic and "in charge" of things—this is not true! When a caregiver refuses support, it may not be due to a lack of caring, but to feeling uncomfortable. When asked about their experiences, most men with partners who have cancer will readily describe being deeply distressed by their partners' illness.

A similar stereotype may be held about women in that they may be perceived as "natural caregivers" who don't need help themselves. This is well described by cancer researcher Laurel Northouse, R.N., Ph.D., who noted, "Nobody brings casseroles to women when their husbands are sick because people assume a woman can do the caretaking. But women need help, too." When compared with men, research suggests that some women may be more likely to complain of physical symptoms—such as back and neck pain, or headaches—in response to the stress of having a partner with cancer. Whether they occur in men or women, these kinds of physical complaints may be a sign of tension that needs to be addressed.

What helps partners cope with the stress of an ill loved one? There is evidence from research studies that people cope better with stress when they have or find supportive people in their lives. For example, some research suggests that married people, on average, adjust better to the stress of a chronic illness than single people. There is some evidence that married people have somewhat better physical and emotional health than single people. Based on these findings, improving the quality of close relationships is worthwhile for all of us, especially during stressful times such as coping with cancer.

Strong family bonds can help buffer emotional distress. We saw this in the case of Yvonne and Bob who remained close throughout Bob's illness and treatment. The support he received from Yvonne made the experience more bearable. Even though he suffered through several hospitalizations, he knew he could rely on Yvonne to be there through "thick and thin."

In the next chapter, we'll explore in more detail how caregivers can cope with partner's cancer diagnosis and treatment and how you can help your partner and your family get through the experience of cancer.

Other Stressors

Financial Costs

In addition to the psychological costs of an illness like cancer, there are significant financial losses. As many as one-fourth of primary caregivers give up or lose their jobs, and approximately one-third of all families lose all of their savings or their major source of income. The recent trend of patients leaving the hospital to go home sooner increases both financial and caregiving demands on both members of a couple. Even those caregivers who continue working may have a loss of income due to absences from work or changing to a lower-paying job.

Social Costs

When a caregiver is forced to give up a job to care for a partner at home, more than just income is lost. He or she also gives up career mobility, advancement potential, and the support network of coworkers and friends. Sometimes going to work can be a relief to a burdened caregiver who needs a diversion from the stress of his or her partner's illness. Because caregivers are immersed in taking care of their ill partners (and children, in many cases), they may become isolated from their friends and other supportive people and enjoyable activities. Even if the healthy partner has the time and energy for a social life, he or she may feel it is inappropriate to have a social life without his or her ill partner being part of it.

Understanding What Your Partner Is Experiencing

Much more has been researched and written about cancer patients than their partners, so in this book, we emphasize the less frequently discussed topic of cancer's impact on the healthy partner. Nonetheless, it is important to provide an understanding of what the partner with cancer is experiencing. Later, we will discuss the psychological effect of having specific types of cancer.

So what is it like to go through cancer? Typically, the initial reaction to the diagnosis is shock, followed by a period of strong emotions, which often include despair, fear, anger, sadness, and guilt. Deciding between the treatment options can be difficult and confusing. Simply learning about all of the treatment options with a new diagnosis of cancer can be overwhelming, and it is daunting to think about undertaking a treatment with potentially unpleasant or even life-threatening side effects. Cancer patients and their partners must break the news of the cancer to the family. It can be confusing to figure out how to present the information to children of differing ages. Some time following the diagnosis patients often begin to confront the possibility of their own mortality. Coming to grips with the possibility of dying takes time, emotional energy, and reflection.

Patients have to adjust to the physical and lifestyle changes brought on by their cancer treatments. Depending on the treatment and patients' responses, hair loss, fatigue, nausea, weight loss, and changes in sexual desire or functioning are some of the potential obstacles faced by patients and families. Changes in household members' roles are often required to allow patients to focus on their treatment regimen.

Even after cancer has been successfully treated, survivors often think about and fear recurrence. Some spouses and loved ones no longer see cancer as a threat, so they may not be prepared for the survivor to stay focused on cancer after treatment is successful. The person with cancer sees life differently after the experience, no longer feeling "immune" to serious illness. In other ways, too, the person with cancer may have a changed outlook or philosophy. This can be difficult for loved ones, who often expect the survivor to be their "usual self." The pain these changes can cause in relationships is one of the major focuses of this book. It offers couples information to better understand what is happening to them psychologically during and after the physical confrontation with cancer.

Specific Cancers and Their Psychological Impact on Couples

While we can make some general statements about cancer and its impact on couples, each type of cancer may involve special challenges. We have devoted the next section to the unique problems involved with each type of cancer. Although we will discuss many possible cancer symptoms and treatment side effects, not all of these will apply to your situation. Your doctor can provide you with the most accurate and specific information about what symptoms, response to treatment, and side effects you may expect. We will discuss all of the many possible complications and problems because they give an idea of the stresses that couples may face when confronting each type of cancer.

Brain Tumors

A diagnosis of a brain tumor is universally stressful for patients and their families. Brain tumors can potentially affect thinking and behavior, and this is frightening for patients. Patients often fear losing control. When patients do develop thinking or behavior changes, it can be extremely stressful both for them and their loved ones. For example, some patients may develop difficulty speaking or understanding what others say, leading to frustration and, of course, sadness for them and partners or family members. Confusion and memory loss are always especially painful for loved ones, who naturally want to talk with the patient about shared memories. A change in your loved one's behavior is a tremendous loss. One specialist's observation of people with brain tumors suggests that the stress of this may cause a crisis in some marriages. If you think your marriage may be in a crisis and you need support to cope with it, refer to Chapter 12 and the *Resource Guide* at the end of the book.

Head and Neck Cancer

One of the particular downfalls of this type of cancer is the changes that may occur in patients' physical appearance after head and neck surgery. Some patients report feeling less attractive and confident. To make matters worse, having these feelings can cause patients to avoid seeing other people whose company they would otherwise take comfort in and enjoy. Also, losing the ability to have some sensations after treatment for head and neck cancer impacts the person's enjoyment of things such as food and physical intimacy. There may be changes in the patient's ability to speak. Other patients may develop difficulty with eating, affecting their nutrition and energy level.

Facing all of these changes and their psychological and social impact can increase the risk for depression and anxiety. Because patients with head and neck cancers seem to be more likely to become suicidal than patients with other types of cancer, it is important for healthy partners to notice changes in the patient's mood or behavior. If your partner is coping with this type of cancer and seems down, ask about how he or she is feeling. Sometimes caregivers may become so focused on helping the patient eat that this replaces other ways of being close, such as shared activities, touching, or conversation.

Finally, if one or both partners suspects that smoking or drinking alcohol may have played a role in causing the cancer, this can stir up strong feelings of anger and/or guilt, which are particularly difficult to deal with during the crisis of an illness. We will talk more about how to cope with anger and guilt in Chapter 5. For now, it may help to know that if this applies to your situation, you are not the first person to feel angry (or guilty) when dealing with cancer.

Gastrointestinal Cancer

Few functions of the body feel as personal and private as that of bowel function. In cancer that occurs in the stomach, intestines, or rectum, there are numerous physical and psychological challenges. The unpredictability of bowel function and problems with gas and diarrhea can cause embarrassing social situations for the person with gastrointestinal cancer. Consequently, many patients with this type of cancer may avoid being with other people, losing an important source of enjoyment and support. In both men and women, sexual functioning may be affected by the surgeries to treat this type of cancer.

People who have stomas (an opening made by surgery to allow elimination of body waste) may be especially likely to have emotional distress and negative feelings about their bodies. As with head and neck cancers, people dealing with the bodily problems of this type of cancer often describe having negative feelings about themselves that affect their relationships with others.

So it is important for family members to be aware of changes in how the patient behaves or seems to be feeling. In Chapter 5 we will talk more about how couples deal with depression.

Lung Cancer

The physical problems that come with lung cancer can affect the patient's emotional well-being, which in turn affects the couple relationship. Fatigue and shortness of breath are common symptoms in lung cancer and its treatment. If the cancer spreads (metastasizes) to the brain, it can cause problems in thinking and memory.

As with other cancers in which tobacco use is thought to play a role, some lung cancer patients are burdened by feelings of guilt about their tobacco use and the idea that they may have played a role in causing their own cancer. Spouses may feel equally resentful about their partner's past or present smoking behavior. As we noted earlier, feelings of anger and guilt are especially painful to have in the context of an illness, but they are not uncommon.

Bladder Cancer

With bladder cancer, it is sometimes necessary to have a surgical removal of the bladder (called a radical cystectomy) and the addition of a stoma (opening) created for urine diversion. After this surgery, some men may have trouble achieving or maintaining an erection. Both of these complications of treatment can affect not only the patient's physical sexual functioning but also his feelings about his body and attractiveness.

For women, a radical cystectomy also involves removal of the uterus (hysterectomy) and ovaries (oophorectomy), and surgical alteration of the vagina. In addition to going through the hormonal changes associated with menopause, women may have some genital pain during intercourse as a consequence of the surgery. Infertility (a consequence of removal of the uterus and ovaries) can also impact both members of a couple emotionally and financially, as well as physically (see Chapter 11 to learn more about coping with infertility).

Male Cancers

Testicular cancers occur in young men, at an age when they are expected to be sexually active and fertile. While removal of the testicles does not physically impair sexual functioning, men may feel self-conscious about their appearance after surgery, and these feelings may psychologically affect sexual response (see Chapter 5 to learn more about concerns related to sexuality).

The potential adverse effects of treatment for prostate cancer often seem devastating to the male patient and his partner. The possibility of incontinence and impotence as a complication of treatment makes patients feel especially anxious when deciding on a course of treatment.

Female Cancers

Gynecological Cancers

Cancers of the uterus, ovary, cervix, and vagina can cause feelings of shame and embarrassment simply because the sexual organs are involved. A woman may also have painful feelings about such issues as loss of fertility, sexual changes, a sense of isolation, or learning of poor chances for recovery in some types of cancers. A woman may prematurely go through hormonal changes that are experienced during menopause, and there are other physical changes with radiation and surgery. Women with cervical cancer may learn that their cancer is possibly associated with the human papilloma virus (a sexually transmitted virus); as a consequence, some patients may think over their sexual history and feel guilty about past sexual behavior. With these losses and worries, women may find intimacy with their partners more difficult, or even unappealing.

Breast Cancer

Watching thirty minutes of television is all it takes to recognize the value our culture places on women's breasts as a symbol of health, beauty, and sex appeal. Losing a breast to cancer or even having a tumor surgically removed from the breast (lumpectomy) and radiation causes lifelong changes in a woman's perception of her body and sexuality. The psychological impact of having breast cancer has been more thoroughly explored than other types of cancer because of its prevalence and the resulting public interest and demand for research and information.

Research suggests that women with breast cancer may somehow get the idea that they have brought on their breast cancer themselves by having a "bad attitude" or not taking care of themselves. These ideas may be particularly difficult for women who have been told such things about themselves before the cancer. If the woman's "attitude" or self-care have previously been the "hot topics" of arguments between the patient and her partner, they can be fueled by the cancer. Women with breast cancer are also especially worried about passing on the risk of breast cancer to their daughters.

Finally, as with gynecological cancers, women may undergo premature menopause with breast cancer treatment. The couple therefore experiences both physical and psychological losses. Pain, fatigue, anxiety, and changes in body image are common themes raised by breast cancer patients. Healthy partners may feel equally upset about many of the same issues as the patient.

Leukemias and Lymphomas

Leukemias and lymphomas are cancers of the blood system. They are often fatal if untreated, and awareness of this can raise distressing concerns for patients. Treatment often requires lengthy hospitalizations, so dependence on family and others is often necessary. The intensive chemotherapy regimens can impact a person's appearance and ability to function. Infertility may result, as well as weight loss, hair loss, and skin changes. Relationships can be tremendously stressed by these disruptive consequences of leukemia and lymphoma treatments.

HIV-Related Cancers

Cancers related to the human immunodeficiency virus (HIV), which causes acquired immunodeficiency syndrome (AIDS), can raise a number of psychological issues. Depression is common, and anxiety disorders (such as phobias and panic disorder) are reported in as many as one-quarter of those with HIV. Anxiety may be worsened by patients' worry about attending to, and remembering, all of the details necessary to follow self-care regimens for an HIV-related illness. Medicines must be taken on a strict schedule, and check-ups must be regular.

In addition to anxiety and depression, some people have problems with their thought processes (cognitive problems) because of illnesses related to

HIV, and when this occurs, the resulting confusion may contribute to feeling anxious and/or depressed. When this happens, it is usually due to lymphomas that are caused by HIV and arise in the central nervous system.

Fear and misunderstandings about HIV persist despite recent treatment advances that have resulted in longer survival. The social pressures resulting from widespread fear and ignorance can contribute to stress in couples coping with HIV-related cancers.

Coping Styles

An important element in coping with a specific type of cancer is understanding what to expect from the illness, the treatment, yourself, and your partner. Everybody has his or her own coping style, so thinking about how you usually function in a crisis—separately and together—can help forestall surprises.

Some couples, for example, deal with difficulty in their personal lives by throwing themselves into their jobs or hobbies and becoming less available to each other. Although this style may help them escape their distress, it can be misunderstood as uncaring. Others, in order to manage their own anxiety, attempt to take control of all information gathering and decision making, thereby leaving the person with cancer with little voice.

In some couples, crisis can cause fighting and blaming (see Chapter 5 to learn more about conflict styles). Some draw closer to one another, perhaps feeling more of a sense of purpose than when life returns to normal. Some reach out to others for support, whereas others draw in and away from the outside world.

Common Dilemmas

Understanding how your partner copes with crisis may help you plan for cancer's effects on family life. Confusion, anger, frustration, anxiety, guilt, or depression can result from any or all of the following.

Role Changes

Almost invariably after a diagnosis of cancer, one partner has to take over the duties of the person who is ill. Over time, the new responsibilities, on top of what may already be a full load, can be a great burden. The couples that seem to adapt best have always been flexible about who does what (see Chapter 4 to learn more about how good relationships function). When both partners have worked and shared household chores, by design or necessity, they have probably had to learn how to fill in for one another. But in those couples in which each partner has a specific, fixed role and the boundaries rarely overlap—such as those with the tradition that the man works and the woman keeps house—the adjustment is likely to be more difficult.

Shifting the balance of power can be trying too. Frequently, one person in the couple is the decision maker, or the one on whom everybody relies in a crisis. So when illness strikes this dominant individual, life can be chaotic while everybody tries to sort out who's "in charge." But it can ultimately bring a couple closer when the other partner is allowed to demonstrate his or her competence.

For most people, self-esteem is defined at least in part by the roles they fulfill in life. For the family member who is sick, giving up these roles even for a short time can be an enormous loss. It may be possible to exchange some responsibilities—trading the bill paying for the lawn mowing, for example—to allow the person with cancer to feel useful while taking some of the load off those who have been picking up the slack.

Disruption of Routines

Most people follow fixed routines in their daily lives, patterns that provide structure and predictability. But when cancer is diagnosed, these usual ways of doing things are thrown up in the air. Everyone has to accommodate the demands of the illness and the treatment schedule, yet at the same time, each person has daily responsibilities that may conflict with the needs of the person with cancer.

Plans for the Future

Every couple has dreams and hopes at every stage of life. Perhaps one of the most difficult coping challenges, therefore, is accepting a future that has suddenly become unpredictable, in which all that you've worked for or dreamed about may not come true—at least not in the way you had hoped or within the time frame you had set. Rather than concentrate on what hopes may be lost, for the time being try to manage by setting new short-term goals and making plans for the near future. You can continue to add steps to the plan as the course of the illness and the potential for recovery become clearer.

An illness that threatens your ability to pursue important personal goals—such as new career responsibilities or retirement plans—tests the strength of relationship bonds. To resolve this potential crisis, try to avoid all-or-nothing solutions, such as forfeiting plans forever. There may be a way to negotiate a temporary compromise with your partner when needs clash.

Relationship Conflicts

Couples who have forgotten how much they mean to one another may be brought closer together by the experience of cancer. But it can also be the straw that breaks the camel's back: Relationships that were deeply troubled to begin with may not survive. Conflicts and problems that existed before the illness could get worse. Much depends on your individual and collective style of functioning. Stress can bring out the best or worst in people, and usually both. Similarly, it reveals the strengths and vulnerabilities in any relationship. Later in this book we'll explore conflict styles and ways to resolve problems through contracts and improved communication.

The Role of Ethnicity and Culture in Coping Styles

In understanding your relationship and the way each of you reacts to the cancer experience, it is helpful to reflect on the heritage you both bring into the relationship. Of course, your personal history includes a lot of individual experiences that aren't easily summarized by your ethnic identity, such as the family you were raised in. Here, we visit the issue of ethnic differences because there is some research available concerning this topic. You may find this a useful starting place for considering other differences in your individual histories that don't relate to ethnic identity.

The influence of your ethnic and cultural background may be particularly important to consider if you and your partner are from different backgrounds. Different cultures may emphasize different ways of coping with illness, stress, and expressing emotions. For example, some cultures may emphasize the extended family, and if you grew up in this sort of environment, you may prefer to turn to relatives as a way of coping with the stress of cancer. If this differs from your partner's background, it can lead to disagreements about whom to include for support while dealing with cancer. If your partner was not raised to make use of that type of sharing, involving the extended family may feel like an invasion of privacy.

Religious practices can also differ between partners. For example, if one of you is not religious and the other prays daily, there may be a clash in coping styles. Some cultures and families may emphasize being "stoic" and keeping emotions private, while others may be used to openness and self-expression during times of emotion. Viewed through the lens of one's own experience, one partner may see the other as "unfeeling," or on the flip side, as "overly dramatic."

Many cultures and religions place importance on personal responsibility for things that happen, and this can influence individuals' reactions to being diagnosed with cancer. In addition, while some cultures may value unquestioning respect for medical professionals, other historically persecuted groups may have learned to fear or mistrust medical professionals as authority figures, who have been untrustworthy in the past.

Although we've focused on ethnicity and culture in this section, we recognize that sometimes the most important differences between partners are individual and not cultural. In either case, it is easy to see how the different backgrounds each partner brings to the relationship can be even more noticeable during a time of stress. You and your partner may have learned different ways of coping (whether individual or cultural), but both of you didn't know about this "culture clash" until it was brought out by the stress of cancer. When such clashes develop, couples struggle to find common ground where both partners are comfortable. When common ground and mutual respect are established, relationships with such richness of traditions, perspectives, and experiences can be especially rewarding.

Chapter Two

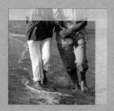

The Caregiver's Role

W e have seen some of the ways cancer affects couples and how cultural and family backgrounds can influence coping styles. In this chapter, we continue to set the stage by taking a closer look at the unique role that caregivers play.

How Caregivers Feel

When I first found out my husband had kidney cancer, I just couldn't believe it. It seemed impossible. He was so young and healthy. Gradually I adjusted to the reality of it, seeing how down he looked, and how sick he felt. It was obvious that he wasn't his old self. Right now I have so much to do. I sometimes just try not to think about what's really happening. It's the only way I can keep going.

This description of the cancer experience illustrates many of the issues that partners of people with cancer typically face. As we mentioned in the first chapter, the person with cancer and the healthy partner may have very similar reactions to the diagnosis. First comes complete shock, often with some denial or a feeling of unreality. Later, the initial disbelief and numbness thaw into emotions such as fear, anger, and sadness. Yet caregivers often feel it is necessary to keep these feelings in check, so that they can function in their new role as their ill partner's advocate, problem-solver, and soother.

Meanwhile, the person with cancer may gratefully refer to their healthy partner as "my rock," without meaning to minimize the partner's feelings. Thus, in the struggle to cope with the cancer diagnosis and treatment, both people may unwittingly fail to acknowledge the impact of the stress on the healthy partner. The aim of this chapter is to help couples better address the caregiver's needs. We will describe the emotional reactions caregivers may typically experience, as well as ways caregivers can take care of themselves emotionally during this stressful time.

As the caregiver, you may watch your partner openly grieve about the cancer while you struggle inwardly with your own painful feelings. It's hard to do both at the same time. Caregivers often listen supportively, allowing their partners to vent their grief and anger. There is a point at which it can start to feel overwhelming for the couple to cope with both partners' strong feelings at once. In order to refuel, you may occasionally need to take a "vacation" from one another. For example, Bonnie and Fred used such a strategy:

FRED WAS MORE EMOTIONAL THAN BONNIE, it seemed—even though he was not the person with cancer. When Bonnie felt as though she was getting more anxious from listening to Fred's fear and sadness over many weeks, she planned a weekend away with her kids. When she came back after several days, she felt more able to respond sympathetically and affectionately to Fred.

Both partners need to talk about what they are feeling. Yet even in the best relationships, people don't have unlimited emotional resources. This means that there are bound to be times when realistically you don't feel up to being a sounding board for your partner. You can let your partner know this as gently and simply as, "My nerves feel exposed. I think I'm feeling too upset myself to talk about this anymore right now, but I promise we can talk again later." That way, the partner in need of support can call a family member or friend until his or her partner feels ready to listen again.

Whether you are the caregiver or the partner with cancer, you'll need to respect yourself and your needs and limits as well as seek support from others.

During the experience with cancer, caregivers often make the mistake of expecting to shoulder all of cancer's many burdens without ever feeling sad or needing support for themselves. But this simply isn't humanly possible. For this reason, it is essential that the healthy partner make contact with other people who can.

The Many Tasks of the Caregiver

Obtaining Information

Over the course of your partner's illness, you will need a great deal of information to help your partner and family cope with the illness. It may help to know that health professionals see it as an important part of their job to respond to your questions. Here are several essential pieces of information you will need:

- First, you'll need an understanding of the illness. What is the diagnosis? What type of cancer is it? Has the cancer spread? If so, how far (what stage)?
- Second, you'll need an idea of what needs to be done. What will you need to know to help your partner decide on a course of treatment? What will you need to do to help with the treatment regimen?
- Finally, you'll need some guidelines about when to call for professional help. What symptoms require immediate attention? If you feel the situation is an emergency and you cannot get the information you need, then call the doctor or an emergency room. Be sure that the person with whom you're speaking understands that you feel this is an emergency.

You'll get the most complete and accurate information by phrasing your questions clearly and knowing exactly what information you need. It may help to write your questions down. Because each member of the health care team has a different function, you may need to ask who is best able to answer each of your questions. If the answer doesn't make sense, or you still don't know how to proceed, be persistent. Don't be afraid to rephrase or repeat your question.

Workplace Issues

Work is often disrupted by the job of taking care of your ill partner and your family. It is reasonable to make your partner your highest priority throughout his or her treatment, but you may still feel badly about missing work or asking coworkers to fill in for you.

The best way to approach work-related issues is to discuss potential problems before they arise. Talk with your boss about your situation. Tell him or her what help you will need and for how long. Be prepared to reopen the conversation with your boss whenever there are new developments in your partner's treatment and condition, updating him or her about unexpected changes or events. Some employers support their coworkers by actually donating extra time off if necessary. Realize, however, that your employer can only help if you honestly communicate your needs up front.

If you are a dual-career couple (see page 192), you may also be able to play a vital role in maintaining your partner's ties to his or her employer. The person with cancer may need a spokesperson or advocate to speak with his or her employer or coworkers about the medical situation. As with your own employer, it is best to be honest and flexible in such conversations.

You may also need to help your partner figure out when and how to return to work. Because you probably know your partner's physical and emotional condition better than anyone else, you may be the person best able to help him or her make a realistic plan.

Talking to Your Children

Most couples share the task of telling their children about the cancer diagnosis. However, the caregiver is most likely to be called upon to answer follow-up questions. Because you are the well parent, your children may feel more comfortable asking you questions that they might hesitate to ask the parent with cancer. Sometimes, these questions may arise at inconvenient times, such as when you have many things to take care of, or when you are feeling particularly sad or anxious. But providing this information to your children is among the most important things you will do as the caregiver. In this section, we provide an overview of some of the main issues, but we address these in greater detail in Chapter 7 (pages 111–117, *Parenting and Cancer*).

Children need to know the truth about what is happening. If they are not told the truth, they may realize this and in their uncertainty imagine that the situation is even worse than it is. Moreover, trying to conceal the situation takes a great deal of effort and energy. This energy is better spent helping the children be fully prepared for the changes that will take place in the family.

In general, children need a clear idea of what their parent with cancer will go through and how it will affect their lives. Present the information simply, at an appropriate age level, and without an overwhelming amount of detail. They need to know about side effects that they will notice, and they need to understand that the parent with cancer may feel grouchy and sick at times.

Here are some suggestions about how to give children information they can understand:

- Explain what has happened.
- Tell them they did not cause the cancer.
- Tell them what will happen next.
- Leave them with feelings of hope that even though everyone is upset, there will be better times to come.
- Assure them they will continue to be loved and cared for.

Listen to how your children respond to the information you are giving them. Then attempt to respond to each child's needs. For example, a six-year-old may fear she can "catch" the disease, while a teenager may talk about feeling embarrassed by the attention that the situation causes with his teachers or peers.

You may want to take your children to see the ill parent in the hospital. A visit to the parent with cancer can reassure children that they are not being abandoned by either parent. However, it helps to prepare them for what they might see when they visit the hospital. You and your partner will also need to discuss your roles and how they may change as a result of the illness. It can help if the ill parent stays as involved as possible with the children, and sometimes your job as caregiver is to ensure that connection is maintained.

You may also need to speak with teachers and other adults at school. School personnel do not need to know details of the illness and treatment, but they need an idea of what the children are going through and how it may affect their lives at school. That way, they can be alert to any problems or changes in the children's behavior.

Maintaining the usual routine is often left to the healthy parent. Most children thrive on structure and routines. During an illness such as cancer, it is difficult at best to maintain family life as usual. Although life will not be the same, you may want to make a concerted effort to keep in place certain activities that will be the same for your children. That will help ease their anxiety and uncertainty.

The actual amount of time you spend with your children is not as important as the quality of time you spend with them. Consider what activities are the most important and what is realistic for you to do. Give highest priority to the most important activities that you're still able to do, such as reading with your children, helping with homework, and playing games. Doing something alone with each child on occasion can make him or her feel special.

One way of taking care of yourself and your children is learning how to set consistent limits. You may not have been the disciplinarian before your partner's illness, and when everyone is under stress, it is tempting to forget about discipline. But this will not ultimately help your children. Taking the time to set or maintain rules and reinforcing them consistently in a clear, loving, and firm manner helps children feel safe, and will allow their behavioral and intellectual development to stay on track.

Coordinating Care

It is challenging for anyone to negotiate today's health care system, and the health care network is particularly complex for people with cancer and their families. One woman whose husband had been diagnosed with cancer remarked, "One day I feel like a nurse, the next day I feel like a traffic cop. Then all of a sudden I'm a social worker!"

Caregivers usually handle much of the scheduling, medication delivery, transportation, and other practical aspects of the treatment process. These ongoing activities are crucial to maintaining a consistent regimen of care for the patient. For example, if you and your partner have a set schedule of pain medication that treats the pain yet keeps the patient alert, you'll want to ensure that this schedule is maintained while in the hospital.

To minimize disruptions for your partner, you'll need to make sure the different experts in oncology care know each other and the treatment plan. You will often be able to help "fill in any blanks" by providing any needed information to the radiation oncology team and the medical oncology team. Your goal is to maintain helpful procedures and routines with minimal disruption as the person with cancer moves from one treatment setting to another.

Keeping track of your partner's need for personal care, special equipment, diet, and enjoyable activities is useful. Even helping your partner communicate worries or concerns to the treatment team can be helpful. Here are some more specific suggestions for coordinating care:

- Plan a consistent medication schedule.
- Give a list to the appropriate medical staff of the names and times of day that medicines are given.
- Write down any special form the medicine is given in (such as liquid or crushed).
- Inform staff of any allergies or sensitivities to medicines or food.
- List any food or beverages that the person prefers.
- Ask the staff for help with problems.
- Identify the need for any special equipment.
- Bring familiar items from home to your partner, such as the mail or the newspaper, while he or she is in the hospital.
- Bring any relaxing music or movies that your partner would enjoy.
- Make sure your partner has clothing that he or she prefers.
- Bring special pillows or sleeping aids if needed.

Sometimes you may worry that you are *too* involved in the care of your loved one. You may hesitate to offer suggestions because you don't want to offend the staff. Most staff will actually appreciate having information that allows them to individualize the patient's care and will encourage your involvement. Helping them learn more about the patient ultimately enables them to provide the best, most personalized care.

Where to Get More Help

There is a wide range of psychological, social, and practical support services available for families with cancer such as:

- Financial assistance or counseling
- Individual counseling or psychotherapy
- Family therapy

- Group support, education, and therapy
- Home care services
- Transportation services

Taking advantages of these services can help you to cope with the stress of the cancer experience and to spend more quality time with your partner throughout the treatment process. We will talk more about some of these services in Chapter 12.

Adjusting to Changes in Your Partner

As your partner goes through the many physical and psychological changes that often accompany treatment for cancer, you as the caregiver must adjust to those changes. Sometimes that adjustment can be painful and complicated. Simply seeing your loved one in discomfort or pain for long periods of time can be a difficult experience for a caregiver. It can leave you feeling powerless and helpless while you try to put on a brave face.

Reactions to physical changes in a loved one can be confusing. We tell ourselves, "The most important thing is what's inside." While there is much truth to this cliché, it is still an adjustment when a loved one's body changes. After all, we have physical relationships with our intimate partners. For example, if your partner loses a breast to cancer, you also experience a loss. At the same time, you fear upsetting her by reacting to the change, so you try to stay as positive as possible. You might feel as though you have to "shut off" your own emotional response to the loss. But having a reaction of sadness to a change in your partner's body does not mean that you love him or her any less. It is natural to have these feelings. Like any other loss, you and your partner may both go through a gradual healing process. As you adapt to the change, your feelings about it will become less intense.

Even as you are having these strong emotional responses, you may feel you're expected to give physical nursing care while also taking care of the household, your job, and your mutual family and friends. Although you do have to keep track of many things, pretending to *feel* strong all of the time can actually be a disservice to your relationship, as well as to your own well-being.

Your partner will want to continue to have a full relationship with you. This can include being your companion, comforter, and friend.

Believe it or not, offering your partner the opportunity to serve in these roles may help your partner's morale and connection with you more than anything else you can do. Your partner may not always respond well to the feelings you share, but this may have been true before the cancer. It is important, nonetheless, to share your feelings whenever and in whatever way feels appropriate to you. Sharing your own feelings of loss or sadness lets your partner know that you still love and need him or her just as much as you ever did, despite the illness.

Most importantly, be yourself and try not to worry about whether you are doing things right. Let your words and your actions come from your heart. Your compassion and genuine caring are the most important things you can convey to your loved one right now.

Caregiver Guilt

As you go through the many tasks, emotions, and challenges of being your partner's caregiver and significant other, you may have some surprisingly strong feelings of resentment, frustration, and even anger. It is natural to feel angry that your partner has cancer, that your life has been completely disrupted, and that you must now carry most of the load. Allow yourself to express those feelings with other people you trust (especially people who are nonjudgmental).

For some, the guilt that goes with the inevitable feelings of resentment can be overwhelming. You may feel awful that you resent your partner for being sick. So you beat yourself up for not having the "right" attitude about what is happening.

You can acknowledge such guilt, anger, and frustration when it comes up, and then let it go. Realize that it is a normal part of the process and will eventually go away. Save your energy for the many important things you need to do for yourself and your partner.

Communication Tips for Caregivers

Keeping an open line of communication can help couples work through the tough times. The following suggestions are designed to help caregivers communicate with their partners. (See the workbook, *Couples' Corner*, at the end of this book for more exercises.)

❧ Let your partner with cancer take the lead. If he or she wants to talk, be a good listener. Listen to what is said and how it is said. It's only natural to talk too much when you feel nervous, but try to get more comfortable with silence. It may help the person with cancer to focus their thoughts. Sometimes silence is comforting.

❧ Try to maintain eye contact so your partner will know that you are being straightforward and open. Touching, smiling, and looks that convey affection show your partner that even though he or she is ill, you care for him or her as you always have.

❧ Try to avoid giving your partner advice while he or she is upset or in shock. Often people give advice because they think it is the only way to be helpful, but advice may be the last thing he or she needs. It may be more helpful simply to ask questions or listen. You, too, may feel more relaxed if there isn't pressure to come up with solutions all of the time.

❧ Try asking your partner how he or she feels rather than saying, "I know how you feel." This will give him or her a chance to talk about the feelings.

❧ If you feel emotional and are having difficulty maintaining your composure, tell your partner what you're feeling, rather than turning away or trying to hide your reaction.

❧ People with cancer do not always want to think or talk about their disease. Laughter and talking about other things are often welcome diversions. This may be too much to ask during the initial shock of the diagnosis, but be watchful that your initial shock doesn't develop into prolonged, uninterrupted somberness. For example, some people mistakenly think that being serious all of the time is the only way to respect what your partner is going through. Don't worry, your respect and compassion will be evident; you don't always have to try so hard to show it.

❧ Try to involve your partner in as many shared activities as possible. If you used to play cards, then play cards now! If you used to go to the movies together, continue to do so. This will be healing time together for both of you. (Of course, always consider your partner's stamina when planning these activities.)

❥ Be aware of the physical and psychological affects of the illness, but try to avoid being overprotective. Continue to invite and urge your partner to do things with you and others. Encourage other friends to visit. If they can't visit, ask them to write or call.

Taking Care of Yourself

You may find that visitors' and callers' attention is focused on your partner, even though you are also going through a difficult time. It is only natural that the focus is on the ill partner and his or her medical condition, treatment, and recovery. But after the numerous phone calls inquiring about your partner's condition, you feel like saying, "Hey, what about me? Are you going to ask how I'm doing?" After all, you may now be juggling a full-time job outside the home, all of the home and childcare responsibilities, and much of the responsibility of being supportive to your ill partner and overseeing his or her care.

As the caregiver, you also hold a lot of information that must be communicated to health care staff, so you may often accompany your partner during treatment visits. Delegating tasks to friends and family is helpful, but often the caregiver must make the decisions about the delegation, which is time consuming.

With all of these demands, make sure you take care of yourself, too. Begin by figuring out what you need to do so you don't do more than you have to. Have an open discussion with your partner to take the guesswork out of figuring out what's expected of you.

Sometimes you may take on responsibilities because you assume your partner expects it. But he or she may have other expectations that you don't know. Decide jointly what your partner needs, what you must do, and what may be delegated to other family and friends. Your responsibilities (that is, those that cannot be delegated) should become your top priorities. This can only happen if your partner's needs and decisions about delegating are openly discussed.

Alicia assumes that she must take care of all the home responsibilities that Keith normally handles while he is recovering
from his bone marrow transplant. It's exhausting for her to take on
these responsibilities at the same time as she's taking care of Keith's
health care needs at home. However, she has never discussed this
with him. As it turns out, Keith feels demoralized when he sees
Alicia sweating and doing yard work when he believes he should be
doing it. He would prefer that they hire someone to assist her with
those chores. But Alicia has been so tired and edgy lately, he just
doesn't want to rock the boat by raising this issue. He figures maybe
it makes her feel good to help out.

If Alicia and Keith sat down to discuss this issue, they would see that both of
them could be satisfied. If they had this discussion and hired someone to help,
then Alicia would be less exhausted, and Keith would not have to feel so badly
about his inability to maintain his former responsibilities. They could even set
aside some private time for each other that could help them reconnect.

In addition to raising issues openly with your ill partner, you need to be
able to take care of yourself. This sounds obvious, but many couples find that
caregiver exhaustion and stress may escalate to a crisis if not addressed.

Since her husband has been ill, Yvonne has been trying to
continue her life exactly as she did before. Since she normally
exercises first thing in the morning, she moved her exercise session
up to 5:00 A.M. to fit it in with all of her other daily responsibilities.
Between the stress of her husband's illness and her anticipation of the
early morning alarm clock, she began having a difficult time sleeping.
Trying to function on little sleep began to cause major problems. It
took a minor traffic accident that happened because she was dazed at
the wheel to make Yvonne realize that she needed to reevaluate how
she was managing her current situation. She didn't want to compromise
her exercise schedule since exercising made her feel calmer, so she
negotiated a new work schedule with her employer.

Burnout Alert

Here are some signs of caregiver burnout to watch out for. Some of these signs are, in fact, symptoms of serious clinical depression. At the very least, they may be signs that exhaustion and burnout are taking a toll on your well-being, even if you aren't clinically depressed.

❧ You're exhausted all the time.

❧ You can't fall asleep, sleep restlessly through the night, or get up too early in the morning.

❧ You've withdrawn from friends, and you've lost interest in the activities that used to bring pleasure.

❧ You feel guilty that you're not doing enough or that you don't want to do any more.

❧ You worry that you've lost the feelings you used to have for the person you're caring for—you just feel numb.

❧ You think the only relief you can get right now is from alcohol, drugs, food, or cigarettes.

❧ You don't feel well.

❧ You're sure that nothing good is ever going to happen again.

Caregiver Burnout

Caring for someone who is sick, taking over his or her responsibilities, adapting to new habits and routines, and worrying about what will happen with your partner's cancer can cause fatigue at the very least. Worse, these combined pressures can lead to resentment, guilt, exhaustion, depression, and even physical illness. If you wait for these things to happen, you may ultimately find yourself unable to continue to care for your loved one until you take care of yourself. This condition is often referred to as caregiver burnout.

There are some things you can do to take care of yourself emotionally and physically to keep burnout from happening. Resist feeling guilty for thinking of yourself. Allow yourself private time and space once in a while.

Pay attention to your need for rest, nutrition, and other self-care. You may even need to ask someone else in your life to help take care of you! Recognize your limits, and forgive yourself for not being perfect and for not being able to do more than is humanly possible for your loved one.

You can cope with burnout by doing some of the following things:

- **Reach out to others.** Ask for support from family, friends, neighbors, people in your church or temple, or others who can offer help. There may be times when finding strength is hard, and the situation feels overwhelming. You may feel as if you can't do this all by yourself. If you are comfortable doing so, widen your circle of resources by reaching out to friends, family, or support organizations. These people can help you remember that you're not alone on this journey. They will be there to share your fears, hopes, and personal accomplishments every step of the way. People are often glad to help. If friends or family members are not able to provide support, find others who can. Health care professionals, such as social workers, psychologists, or other licensed health professionals, and support groups are additional sources of support.

- **Delegate, delegate, delegate.** You may need to hand over some of the responsibilities that you think you "should" be able to shoulder by yourself. Ask family members, even those that may be out of town, to help out if possible. Divide responsibilities according to each person's strengths, interests, and personalities. For example, some people are better at dealing with paperwork rather than providing a soothing presence at the bedside. Some may be good at dealing with medical personnel and taking notes, whereas others may prefer to run errands or cook meals. Those who may be unable or unwilling to contribute time might be in a position to help out financially.

- **Build your knowledge base.** Some people find that learning as much as they can about their partner's diagnosis and treatment gives them a sense of control over what happens. Even if you don't want a lot of scientific information, you can find out what has helped other partners cope with cancer, and/or talk with other people who are in a similar situation.

- **Express your feelings.** Many people discover that finding a way to express feelings of sadness, fear, or anger can help them maintain a positive attitude about the cancer process. Some people believe that expressing such feelings is a sign of weakness. In fact, the opposite is often true; it takes courage to express such feelings. Openly acknowledging your feelings allows you to find ways of coping with them. There are many ways to express your feelings; find one that is most comfortable for you and most compatible with your personality and circumstances. You might choose to talk with trusted friends or relatives, keep a private journal, or even try expressing your feelings through painting or drawing.

- **Take time to do something you enjoy every day.** Prepare your favorite meal, spend time with an uplifting friend, watch a movie, meditate, listen to your favorite music, play cards, or do whatever else you find enjoyable. Physical activities such as dance, yoga, sports, and stress reduction techniques can improve your sense of well-being. Poetry, music, drawing, woodworking, and reading are also creative ways to express yourself.

- **Seek spiritual support.** Religious beliefs and activities can be a source of strength for many people. Some cancer survivors and their loved ones find that cancer strengthens their existing faith or that their faith gives them strength. Ministers, rabbis, and other faith leaders, or a trained pastoral counselor, can help you find spiritual support. Some members of the clergy are specially trained to provide counseling to people with cancer and their families. Most hospitals have chaplains available.

- **Distract yourself.** There's no reason to focus all your thoughts on your loved one's illness—in fact, there's every reason not to. Go out for dinner or to the movies. Have a good laugh. Play games with your partner or a friend. Go on a vacation, if only for a day. Remember that if you're able to lighten your mood, you'll take better care of your partner. Your partner may actually feel better knowing that you are taking good care of yourself.

Emotional Health Care

There is a difference between feeling appropriately sad and having serious depression. If the sad feelings go on for weeks without improvement, you may be clinically depressed (see Chapter 5 for the signs and symptoms of clinical depression). Being seriously depressed can greatly interfere with your ability to manage all the tasks of being a caregiver. Depression can continue for a long time if it is not treated. Moreover, depression may feed on itself. Because you feel depressed, you have less energy to put into solving problems. When problems do not get resolved, you feel worse while the actual problems get worse. Even if you think that you can live with your depression, if your depression is not addressed, it may affect your partner as well.

Asking for help in dealing with depression, anxiety, or other emotional concerns is not a sign of weakness, but a sign of effective coping. A professional can help you find useful solutions to the problems that you are facing. Psychosocial services (or supportive care) help people solve problems that involve psychological or social functioning. If you feel your concerns are not being addressed adequately as you go through the first weeks of your loved one's illness, or if you find that you are anxious and depressed as described above, you may need to access psychosocial support services.

In addition to the risk of becoming anxious or depressed, sometimes caregivers have a difficult time talking about the illness and their feelings about it. It is especially hard to talk about feelings of anger and guilt. Sometimes a counselor can help you express these feelings in a safe, nonjudgmental environment.

The availability of support services will depend on where your partner is receiving treatment. In large cancer centers or at universities, services are usually available within the treatment setting. In smaller communities, you may find services from other agencies in the community, private counselors, or support programs (see Chapter 12 for more information about when to seek therapy and how to choose a therapist).

The Gift of Caregiving

There is little doubt that caregiving can be challenging. But it can also be one of the most rewarding things you have ever done. Some people look back on the experience of caregiving as the closest period of their relationship. Some find that they have more strength than they ever imagined. Most caregivers in good relationships find great satisfaction in caring for the person they love most. If your relationship has been a good one, you may feel it is a way of repaying your partner for all of the wonderful things he or she has brought to your life. Even your other relationships may be deepened by the experience of caring for your ill partner.

You may be more aware of how precious life is now, how important you truly are to your partner, and how important he or she is to you. This knowledge can be a precious gift for some people. But if you are struggling right now, your relationship is having problems, or you can't see any silver lining in it all—or even if you're keeping your head above water but could use some more guidance—we hope the following chapters will help.

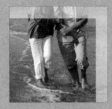

Chapter Three

Evaluating
Your Relationship

To evaluate your own relationship, you will need to understand the general process couples go through in developing and sustaining a relationship, and what key ingredients are involved. It is these factors that may be stretched to the limit when someone is diagnosed with cancer. Here we provide some ideas about how to understand and assess the status of your relationship.

What Makes the Couple's Bond Unique?

Although couples sometimes describe themselves as being "best friends," committed love relationships are not exactly like friendships. The relationship you build with a chosen mate is also different from other family relationships. Here are some of the things that make couples' relationships unique:

- **Couples' relationships are entered into voluntarily.** You can't choose your family, but in our society, you can usually freely choose your mate.

- **Couples' relationships need to be both predictable and flexible.** Partners in a relationship make a commitment to share many aspects of their lives, even when this means stretching to meet each other half way. Although friendships can be predictable, they are often less flexible than committed love relationships (how many fishing buddies would be open to the suggestion of going to the ballet instead?). The same can be said about family relationships. Typically, by the time we reach adulthood, the families we grew up in have long-established traditions. With so many generations having gone before us, it may be hard to "break the mold."

- **Couples' relationships always have a past, present, and future.** Of course, the same can be said of many friendships and family relationships. However, friendships may have a "take it as it comes" quality that is different from the committed quality of a long-term love relationship. We may have a long or a relatively short history with our friends. Family relationships usually have a shared past, but as we get older, we may or may not continue to have the same closeness with members of the family we grew up in.

- **Being part of a couple means supporting each other.** Although support may be an important aspect of some friendships, we may also have friends who mainly serve to satisfy our need for entertainment or companionship. Mutual support and nurturing are not essential ingredients in friendships, as they are in love relationships.

- **Being part of a couple means that each of you have two identities: as a couple and as an individual.** Couples develop a similar sense of shared identity. Having been in a twosome for many years, some couples describe difficulty maintaining their individual selves. They struggle to maintain their individual interests and may have a hard time conceiving of themselves separate from their "other half." Other couples may have difficulty building a shared "couple identity," feeling more comfortable with their old, separate selves.

- **Couples have a shared worldview.** This follows from what we just said. You may have different opinions than your friends and thrive on the lively debates that ensue. We are sure you've had some lively debates with your partner, too! Still, part of the voluntary decision to enter a committed partnership is the creation of common life goals, such as raising a family together, and in this process, lifestyle choices and values usually grow to intersect in important ways.

For all of us, forming a voluntary, equal, intimate partnership is new territory in adulthood, sometimes exciting and sometimes unnerving. In our experiences while growing up, we may or may not have seen optimal examples of love relationships. Because the couple's relationship is universally new, it can take many blind, stumbling forays over uncharted terrain before becoming smooth and rewarding. Now let's examine how couples' relationships typically develop over time.

The Three Phases of Couples' Relationships

Like individuals, couples develop in stages over time. The first stage is best known as the honeymoon phase. This is the time when both partners put their best foot forward. They may feel passionately romantic and see each other in the flattering glow of these feelings. In the ordinary course of events, the transition to the second stage happens gradually. The following story illustrates both the changes that happen during the second stage and how cancer can make these changes more dramatic and abrupt.

DEAN AND MAGGIE HAD ONLY BEEN MARRIED A YEAR when Dean was diagnosed with testicular cancer. They had just purchased a new home and were almost ready to try to have a baby. Things had been great that first year. However, after Dean was diagnosed and began his treatment regimen, their honeymoon phase ended abruptly. Although Dean tried not to be too demanding of Maggie, he found himself becoming more critical of how she did things—it was just so frustrating when he couldn't do things for himself. At the same time, Maggie began to have a hard time seeing this bald, weakened, sometimes miserable person as the attractive, ambitious man she married.

Cancer has a way of crashing into new love and its pleasant and hopeful fantasies with harsh realities. This confrontation is especially difficult for new couples, who may still be in the early bloom of that romantic first stage.

The second stage involves a settling-in period, during which couples begin to work out patterns of relating to each other. Typically, couples enter the second stage gradually, usually by beginning to relax into the relationship, often reverting to their former "single" habits. This may feel like a downhill slide, as some of the care and flexibility of the early relationship seems to decline. Now each partner appears more clearly in focus, as imperfections rise to the surface. In this phase, both members of the couple may feel betrayed as neither proves to be exactly "as pictured" when the relationship was new.

In the third stage, there is often a happy medium as each partner develops a fuller and more realistic understanding and acceptance of the other, which allows both partners to negotiate compromises and accommodate one another's preferences and personalities. They grow to accept, and may even treasure, the differences between them and the closeness that results from fully knowing each other. The process of accepting each other "warts and all" is a delicate balancing act, and some couples may fail to bounce back from the shock and sense of betrayal after seeing each other in a less rosy light. At worst, the ensuing crisis can result in emotional "cold war" or out-and-out separation or divorce.

Rather than proceeding in an orderly sequence, these three stages may come and go throughout the life of a relationship. There may be times when romance is recaptured, and other times when the relationship seems endlessly mundane. In healthy relationships, both partners are flexible enough to accommodate each other's changing needs in a well-coordinated dance, remaining committed to one another and ultimately rising above the hurdles presented during each period of change. Yvonne and Bob (described in the Introduction) seem to show this type of optimal love relationship.

Four "Active Ingredients" of Couples' Relationships

There are many things that couples share, do, and feel. If we distilled an intimate relationship to its essence, what would we find? There are at least four "active ingredients" in couples' relationships: commitment, connection, communication, and sexual intimacy. As we define and explore each of these aspects of relationships, be aware of how they play out in your own relationship.

Commitment

Relationships change and evolve. A solid commitment allows couples to incorporate these changes in positive ways. At a minimum, to commit to a relationship means to promise to stay together no matter what. Optimally, commitment implies a promise to work for the best possible relationship. Both promises are based on the belief that the relationship is valuable enough to invest in and make sacrifices for.

One way that couples make sacrifices in the service of commitment is by setting limits on the role of "outsiders" in the relationship. Often the process of forming a committed relationship indicates to relatives that there is now a boundary line between the "new family" of the couple and the "old families" that each member of the couple grew up in. Each partner should feel that he or she is a priority to his or her partner, and that the relationship is protected to some degree from outside demands and influences on each partner.

What are some other reasons why commitment is essential or necessary? Commitment provides psychological safety and security. A solid commitment allows members of the couple the freedom to live without fear of the other partner leaving when "the going gets rough." Problems with commitment typically surface at times of crisis, such as a cancer diagnosis. When there is a crisis, relationships don't always feel rewarding. A solid long-term commitment allows the couple to ride out these bleak times. Couples rarely discuss their commitment, so it sometimes comes as a shock when the commitment of one or both partners is not strong enough to sustain a major stress.

Commitment comes with other challenges. Couples have the difficult task of balancing the commitment to the relationship on the one hand, with concern for each partner's individual needs on the other. If the right balance is not achieved, it has implications for the couple's ability to cope well with a cancer diagnosis. When one partner is in crisis, the focus may shift from the needs of the couple to the needs of the individual. When relationships are in good "health," the partners are usually able to switch back and forth fairly easily between focusing on the individual and focusing on the couple. In the case of

Alicia and Keith (described in the Introduction), both partners became stuck focusing on their separate struggles, and they were no longer able to work as a team.

Ideally, both partners are equally committed to the relationship. Not surprisingly, relationships are most likely to endure when commitment is very strong and mutual. When commitment is unequal or unsteady, the partners' optimism or pessimism about their commitment can make a difference in the chances of a good outcome. If one partner firmly believes there is no hope of reviving a shaky commitment, it can be difficult to convince the other partner that things *can* improve. Couples have the best chance for success when both partners are committed to working to make their relationship as satisfying as possible.

Connection: Balancing Attachment and Independence

What Is Attachment?

Forming attachments is something we do throughout life. A stable, secure attachment involves both staying close to a particular person who makes us feel safe, and feeling safe enough to leave that person's side for a period of time to explore the outside world independently. As you know, a good sign that you feel attached to someone is your feeling of happiness when you see that person and your sadness when you part. The attachment process also includes the desire for touch, the ability to play and be joyful together, and the ability to respond emotionally to each other's unspoken expressions of emotion.

The ability to form attachments is thought to be important for physical survival, since our safety (especially in childhood) depends upon having other people available for assistance. As adults, attachment is important for sexual closeness and closeness with our own children. There is good evidence that how attached we become to others in adulthood is influenced by early experiences with forming and keeping attachments as an infant and young child. This has special importance for couples because each partner's early experiences with attachment relationships (usually with mothers and fathers) may affect his or her behavior with those to whom he or she feels attached in adulthood.

Attachment is a process that is quite natural and intuitive for people who had dependable attachments in childhood. But if a child is led to believe that his or her parent will not reliably return after a separation, the child may try to prevent separation from occurring in the first place by "clinging" when the parent is present. Similarly, if a child has reason to believe that protection or closeness will simply not be available from an adult (for example, an adult behaves in rejecting ways when closeness is attempted), the child may learn to behave in self-sufficient ways and stop attempting to form attachments to others. It is easy to see how these early learning experiences can affect our behavior in close relationships as adults.

These sorts of early experiences might result in an adult having great difficulty forming attachments or feeling a need to stay close at all times. Some adults with unpredictable early experiences may feel confused, yearning for closeness, but unsure of *how* to form and maintain close relationships. The case of "Mattie" helps to illustrate these kinds of difficulties.

MATTIE WAS HER MOTHER'S FIFTH CHILD. At the time she was born, her mother felt she could not handle a new baby because she still felt overwhelmed by the recent death of her own mother. So the family decided that Mattie would go to live with her paternal grandmother when she was three months old. This arrangement lasted for a year, after which Mattie returned to live with her mother, father, and siblings. As an adult, Mattie noticed that she always felt terrified as soon as she began to feel close to a man. She found that she would end the relationship rather than tolerate this intense sense of dread. After talking about this with a therapist, Mattie realized that the disruptions in her attachments to adults during her childhood had probably played a major role in her fear of becoming attached to someone in adulthood. She was later able to find ways of coping with her fear and ultimately formed a successful long-term relationship.

History Is Not Destiny

Most of us want to know what to expect, and we don't like surprises. People tend to predict the future based on past experiences. To oversimplify a bit, imagine that each early relationship is recorded in your mind like a photograph. If you could mentally average the photographs, it would give you an idea of what your next relationship might look like, how the other person will behave, and how you will feel. Sometimes the current relationship really isn't anything like our "mental picture," and this can cause problems. We may feel and act as if our mental picture is a useful "blueprint" of the current situation, even when it isn't.

ONE OF THE REASONS THAT BONNIE (described in the Introduction) could tolerate Fred's intense displays of emotion during her experience with cancer was because she knew things about Fred's past that helped her make sense of his behavior. During Fred's childhood, his mother was distracted and often didn't seem to pay attention to the children. Fred found out later that his mother had been involved in a financial dispute with her siblings at the time. During those years, Fred found that if he yelled and cried, his mother would finally give him the attention he needed.

As an adult, Fred had not really learned different ways of behaving when things happened to upset him. Fred's mental picture might have included an image of himself, feeling lonely and hungry for attention, and his mother, looking the other way until he started to cry. His unspoken assumption in the present might be, "Unless I'm loud, people I love won't respond." Since Bonnie knew that his behavior made sense based on his earlier experiences, she didn't take it personally and was able to make some allowances for it rather than immediately insisting that he stop complaining, or becoming upset herself. This helped Fred calm down and behave more appropriately.

Early experiences in attachment relationships can affect all aspects of current relationships, right down to selecting a mate. Even someone who swears, "I'll never marry anyone like my mother" may ultimately feel most comfortable with someone who looks like that mental picture. But it is important to realize, especially if you tend to remember mainly painful and disappointing aspects of your early relationships, that early attachment experiences do not fate us to repeat history. A person might select someone who reminds them of only the positive sides of their early attachment figures, while another may select someone who offers qualities that seemed lacking in early attachment figures.

The process of forming a couple can also offer a second chance for people who have had negative attachment experiences in the past. To take advantage of this opportunity, it is helpful if both members of the couple have detached themselves from other (particularly negative) attachments and are able to invest much of their energy in the new relationship. Once in a relationship, people often find that specific behavior in their partner may at times seem to resemble the mental picture of earlier attachment figures, especially parents. Although we focus on negative mental pictures here, it is important to note that the same process happens with happy memories as well.

If you are involved in a current situation with your partner and you get a feeling as if you've been here before—or even if you notice yourself reacting in ways that seem extreme and perplexing to you or your partner—think about how the current situation may resemble earlier experiences. For example, you might have the thought, "This makes me feel just like when Mom ignored me." There are certain times when it is useful to think about how the current situation may resemble your old mental picture of early relationships. For example, sometimes you may notice a sudden rush of intense negative emotion in response to something your partner says or does. You may feel angry, sad, hurt, scared, or ashamed. You may feel that you need to protect yourself by withdrawing, asking for reassurance, or yelling. The feeling you get may seem old and familiar. You may have recurring, intense anger accompanied by a "Here we go again" feeling. Of course, sometimes your reaction may be appropriate to the situation at hand. Still, it is important to be aware of how the old mental picture can influence your reaction to (and interpretation of) events in the present.

Many people in close relationships have times when they feel as if they can read their partner's mind. You've probably had this experience yourself. When this happens to you, and you find yourself making assumptions about your partner's thoughts and feelings, it may be especially important to consider the possibility that you are working under old assumptions from your earlier experiences, or drawing conclusions based on mental pictures from the past. It is helpful to give your partner a chance to confirm or deny your "mind reading" conclusions.

Unfounded fears of abuse or rejection (when there is no evidence whatsoever that these fears are plausible in the current relationship) may also be an indication that earlier experiences are creeping into the present. If there is no sign that your partner has any potential for abusive behavior, yet you still feel extreme fear or panic during a minor conflict that perplexes both you and your partner, it is worthwhile to consider whether your early history could make sense of the perplexing feelings. For example, any kind of conflict can induce this type of panic in people who grew up in violent, extremely unpredictable, or emotionally abusive households. For other people, fears and emotional reactions to conflict may be much milder than this but still out of proportion to the situation.

The general concepts we are discussing go beyond those who were unhappy as children. It is not necessary to "blame" your parents for your current relationship problems in order to consider how your early experiences (and assumptions or expectations developed over time) may have influenced your reactions to things that happen in your current relationship. Once you have recognized a repeated pattern of becoming overly upset or fearful in certain situations that you think may remind you of earlier experiences, you can talk about the reaction with your partner. We will discuss how to handle these sorts of problems in the last section of this book, called *Solutions*.

How Do We Explore Our Strengths and Problem Areas?

By taking the time to explore each other's past experiences with close relationships, you may learn important things about the strengths and weaknesses of your current relationship. If you'd like to have this kind of conversation with your partner, it is important to do it when both of you are calm and not in the midst of an argument (otherwise, you will both be defensive and not in the mood to share details about your past). If there is constant and intense tension between you, these conversations may be best postponed or done with a professional therapist (see the *Resource Guide* at the end of this book). Make sure that you have the time and energy to listen to each other's experiences. Be prepared to be open and not critical. These conversations don't have to be formal affairs or completed in one sitting, but it does help if you are face to face with your partner.

Ask each other about your parents and how close you were with each parent. Offer each other an invitation to talk about your most memorable experiences with each parent. Talk about whether each of you was close to

Questions from the Past

You can learn a lot about your partner and your relationship by asking these questions:

❥ What were your mother and father like when you were young?

❥ How close were you to them when you were little?

❥ What were things like between you and your mother? What about you and your father?

❥ What were things like between your mother and your father?

❥ When you think about your parents, what kind of picture comes to your mind?

❥ Are you close to your siblings?

❥ What was it like when someone in your family got sick?

❥ What was it like when you were sick?

❥ What were important relationship experiences that happened to you as a child? When you were an adolescent?

❥ Do you see any particular patterns in your relationships?

your siblings. Ask about relationship experiences each of you had that seemed particularly important from your childhood, adolescence, and adulthood. Talk about the role that illness played in your family. Tell each other about any "themes" you see in the memories each of you has of prior relationship experiences. (In this conversation, you don't need to point out how these themes relate to your present relationship.)

We suggest that you postpone discussing any current difficulties in your relationship until you read later sections of this book. But it is a good idea to show your appreciation for opening up to each other, and let each other know if you find the information helpful or if it makes you feel closer to your partner.

"Come Closer—No, Go Away!"

It is normal and common for people in close relationships to alternate between wanting distance, independence, or freedom on the one hand, and wanting to be close on the other. Quite frequently, one partner is repeatedly "chasing" his or her mate (in search of closeness, affection, or support), while the other partner repeatedly tries to back off or "get space." The following scenario may sound familiar to some readers.

> TOM'S BEEN FEELING A LITTLE PRESSURED AT WORK, and it really helps to go off by himself and think. Cheryl follows him into the study and asks him to put his book away so they can talk. He's a little torn, and he doesn't answer right away. Cheryl starts to feel upset and she can hear her voice sounding edgy. "Tom, I said I want to talk— what's so hard about that?" Tom again falls silent and then says, "Honey, back off." Cheryl thinks to herself, "We're growing apart." She feels scared. She gets a little bit teary and says, "Tom, why can't you stand to be close to me?" Tom feels guilty, but sometimes it gets on his nerves when she sounds so needy and emotional. He thinks, "Can't she see I'm stressed out and I just need time to myself—is that wrong?" His voice starts to sound angry when he says, "Cheryl, please—there's no need to get upset, I'm just not in the mood to talk right now." She starts to cry harder. Tom says, "I knew this would happen—why do we have to keep doing this?"

A part of relationships involves being independent at times, as well as feeling close and dependent on each other. As you may have noticed, we're not always perfectly "in sync" with our partners where independence is concerned. There are some gender differences, with women being in the role of the stronger "pursuer" (of closeness) slightly more often, and men on average being in the role of the stronger "withdrawer" in the relationship. However, in any given relationship, these roles may be reversed. They may also be reversed when a crisis occurs. For example, a woman who has been diagnosed with breast cancer may withdraw under the stress of her illness.

There is no gold standard for the exact amount of independence, so when we differ with our partners, there isn't a clear right or wrong. For this reason, people feel confused about their need for independence—is it self-reliance (positive spin) or selfishness (negative spin)? They wonder, "Is having independence hurtful to our closeness?" If women find themselves in the traditionally "masculine" position of being the withdrawer in the relationship, they may feel especially uncomfortable being in that role. Some people actually ask their partners for permission to feel more comfortable about having independence.

Relationships are usually most satisfying if there is some flexibility. Relationships work best if both partners have both the ability and the willingness to be close or independent when required, or in response to each other's needs. Flexibility in a relationship is crucial when dealing with cancer because the usual needs will shift throughout the demands of the illness.

Communication: Why and How to Do It

As illustrated by the story of Tom and Cheryl (on the previous page), communication can be verbal (words) or nonverbal (tone of voice and facial expression). Both types of communication can significantly influence the quality of relationships.

Communication serves many important functions, including:
- Expressing feelings
- Communicating practical information
- Receiving information as well as giving it

Good communication enriches relationships, while communication problems can be damaging to relationships. Good communication is much harder than it seems. In mutually satisfying relationships, both partners usually share a range of feelings with each other, and come to some agreement (usually not explicit) about what styles of communicating are comfortable to both partners.

A style that works for one couple may not work for another couple. For example, people differ in how emotionally expressive they tend to be. One cancer survivor fondly referred to her husband's family as the "Loud Family." Although she did not think her husband was particularly loud, she observed that in general, his family yelled up and down the steps to each other constantly. She found this style of communication to be grating. If her husband was from the "Loud Family," she thought she must be from the "Quiet

Family." In her household as a kid, voices were never raised and people stewed about their anger silently without ever expressing it directly. Although she realized that being reserved wasn't always the best way, being more boisterous just didn't feel natural to her. This initially proved to be a challenge for her and her husband in their marriage.

There are many things that determine the intensity of emotional expression that people tend to favor. We mentioned earlier that people who often felt ignored in early relationships may have adapted to this by developing a habit of speaking loudly or repeating themselves. So, some people do this because they don't feel their partner is actually hearing what they want to communicate, even when this may not be the case.

Many communication problems are actually problems that happen on the listener's end. People may focus only on hearing what they want to hear. Listening well is a compliment. It says to your partner, "I care about you and what you have to say. I care about what you are feeling and thinking. You're important to me."

Body language that shows you are listening in a caring way includes:
- Eye contact
- Leaning closer
- Nodding or interjecting yes
- A change in facial expression in response to what the speaker is saying
- An open posture, with arms uncrossed
- Removing or moving away from distractions such as music or reading

Here are some nonverbal and verbal elements of communication that can be harmful. Pay attention and make note if any of the following are present in your relationship:
- Harsh, loud tone or yelling
- Finger pointing, "rolling" of the eyes, or staring
- Sarcastic or patronizing comments (such as "Tell me something I *don't* know!")
- Insults or name-calling
- Statements that often begin with "You did…" (or "You feel/think/are…") rather than "I felt…"

- Referencing sensitive issues when they are not the topic at hand
- Withholding from your partner what you know he or she needs or wants (often this looks like sulking)
- Discussions that are always restricted to superficial or trivial topics
- Interrupting discussion of sensitive issues with anger or prematurely changing the subject
- Making emotional references to other people's relationship problems that parallel your own, without admitting that you are trying to tell your partner something about your own relationship
- Becoming defensive when your partner asks you for your thoughts and feelings
- Changing the topic if asked a question that makes you uneasy
- Repeated reluctance to express your own opinion for fear of angering your partner
- Repeated apologies or, conversely, refusal to forgive
- Rejecting all of your partner's proposed solutions but refusing to suggest your own
- Saying "I don't know," even when you do have something to say (but are avoiding saying it)

Sometimes people develop poor patterns of communication without being aware that they are doing anything wrong. The first step is to identify your communication patterns. We discuss ways to improve communication in Chapter 8.

Reasons for Conflict

Conflict in intimate relationships can be productive if it is motivated by a desire to resolve differences, negotiate compromises, develop solutions to recurrent problems, or convey unexpressed feelings or needs. However, beware when conflict becomes entirely driven by a need to compete for dominance or power. Sometimes the level of competition, which is common in all relationships to some degree, can overcome the spirit of cooperation. When being kind means "losing the game," the spirit of competition has gone too far. When you feel you must always have the upper hand, when you barter rather than discuss, when you feel you must "get credit" for any concession and always have the last word, you are probably focusing more on competition than conflict resolution in your relationship.

Sometimes couples have the same fight over and over again, in slightly different forms. This could be referred to as the "core argument" (see Chapter 6). For example, Mike and Jody argue about spending money on entertainment. She wants cable TV with all the channels and he doesn't. But the issue that they are really fighting about is who has the power within the relationship. Most couples have some recurring themes in their arguments. Having learned more about your partner's family, you may have developed some theories about why each of you focuses on your particular core issue.

The Critical Partner

Some people find fault with their partners to the degree that criticisms become much more frequent than supportive statements. It is difficult to feel comfortable if you are always feeling criticized or not up to the standard of your critical partner. Despite the cliché that self-worth should not be determined by others' evaluations of us, we can't help but find our self-esteem suffering if we are the target of constant put-downs.

People who frequently criticize their partners often seem to have the expectation that their standards for their partner's behavior are more important than their partner's right to be an (imperfect) individual. Although criticisms of people we know well may have a basis in fact, sometimes people are overly critical of others for flaws that they most fear in themselves—self-criticism often goes with being critical of others. In your relationship, do you find yourself or your partner being overly critical? Sometimes the pressure of an illness can bring out the critical side in others.

The Unassertive Partner

Sometimes people become so uneasy with conflict that they take a passive or unassertive approach. Here are some behaviors that may show that there are some problems being direct or assertive:

- Do you listen to what your partner says, agree, but then talk about how it probably won't work?
- Do you act like you don't understand when your partner suggests something that might change the relationship?
- Do you act as though you're not able to do something that you don't want to do?

- Do you suddenly become ill and make excuses to undermine mutual plans?
- Do you find yourself saying often, "Yes, but...?"

Sometimes what we are thinking has nothing to do with what we are actually saying. Let's listen to what Marge and Henry are saying and thinking:

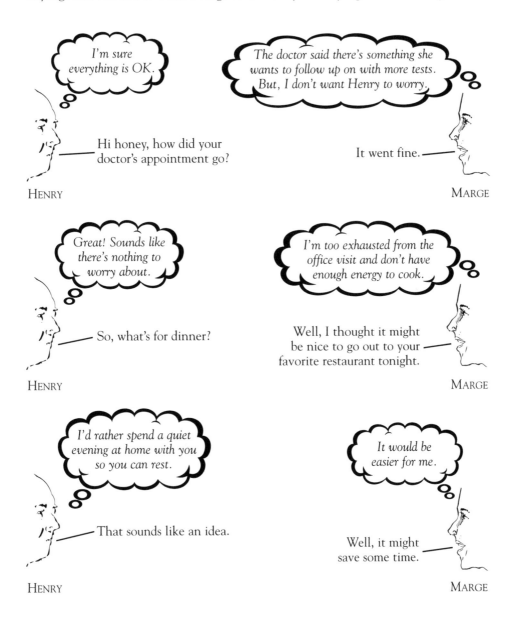

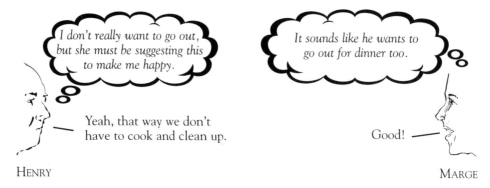

HENRY   MARGE

In this exchange, Marge and Henry don't even come close to expressing what they are thinking or feeling. Sometimes being honest may be harder than it seems, especially when there is tension or anxiety.

Gender and Style Differences

We should be wary of offering generalizations that suggest gender differences are either universal or absolute. Also, it is important for you and your partner to appreciate your different styles of being close whether they are related to your gender or not. The observations of popular self-help writers may offer a starting point for a discussion between you and your partner about your differences. Do you think these observations about men and women are true? Do they apply to your relationship?

In his book, *Men Are from Mars, Women Are from Venus*, John Gray, Ph.D., talks about some style differences often seen in men and women. The following typical style differences are helpful to think about, even if they don't fall neatly along gender lines:

- Talking about problems (women) versus being by yourself to think about problems (men)
- Acknowledging feelings before solving a problem (women) versus doing the problem-solving first (men)
- Wanting to be cherished (women) versus wanting to be needed (men)

Deborah Tannen, Ph.D., author of *You Just Don't Understand: Women and Men in Conversation*, describes the following communication styles:

- Focusing on action (men) versus focusing on connection (women)
- Focusing on mutual cooperation (women) versus challenging your conversation partner or debating (men)

- Focusing on comparison (men) versus focusing on empathy or sharing (women)

We hope that the styles described serve as a starting point for a discussion of the style differences between you and your partner, even if you think that these styles have little to do with your gender—or if you are in a same-sex relationship. When you recognize the language of communication that each of you favors, you can understand the real message in your communications. Differences between you can be not only acknowledged, but actually celebrated. Understanding the style differences between you can lead you to feel closer to each other, which can help you manage cancer together.

Sexual Intimacy

Sexuality can be one of the most emotionally charged issues between partners, and one that many couples find difficult to talk about. Physical intimacy through sexual expression is unique to love relationships. The specifics of optimal sex are different for everyone, and partners generally try to find common ground where both are comfortable and satisfied.

Although there is no rule book for good sex, some general guidelines are helpful, especially because sex is often so private that we may not be comfortable comparing notes with others. Carol Ellison, Ph.D., sex therapist, once said, "You're having good sex if you feel good about yourself, good about your partner, and good about what you're doing. If later, after you've had time for reflection, you still feel good about yourself, your partner and what you did, you know you've had good sex." In the next chapter we discuss what makes a rich and pleasurable sexual relationship, and further on we explain how to strengthen your physical relationship (see Chapter 10).

It is normal and common for conflict and feelings of emotional distance between partners to interfere seriously with the sexual relationship. It is hard to be spontaneous, exposed, and playful when one person is furious with, or— even worse—afraid of, the other. If one partner feels mistreated, neglected, or constantly criticized, it will be difficult for him or her to have sexual feelings or even to feel good. Sometimes even couples who generally have a harmonious relationship may have certain sexual difficulties, such as premature ejaculation or differences in sexual appetite that cause problems in the relationship.

Sexual intimacy often depends on the quality of the couple's emotional attachment. Knowing your partner's body and sexual responses and being emotionally accessible to one another all are part and parcel of the total relationship. Many experts feel that sex and a good emotional connection are inseparable. Having sex and physical intimacy with a person you love is a vulnerable act. It is also a way to give and receive trust, love, and respect. (In Chapter 9, we explain how couples can develop more emotional intimacy.)

The connection between the emotional and sexual components of a relationship means that one of these components may be "contaminated" by problems in the other component. For example, sex may be withheld or doled out in a controlling fashion to punish or manipulate one's partner (but of course, you should always explore your partner's reason for refusing sex *before* making this interpretation). Feeling sexually rejected by one's partner can have a damaging impact on both the relationship and one's self-esteem.

To add to these potential sources of conflict, cancer may have a sudden and unwanted effect on the sexual life of a couple either because of the emotional or physical aspects of the disease and its treatment. (We discuss the impact of cancer on emotions, intimacy, and sexuality in more detail in Chapter 5.)

The quality of a sexual relationship is often difficult for couples to talk about and evaluate together. Avoidance of this subject is common, but once the subject is open, there are often many simple things that can improve sexual communication. Given the connection between emotional intimacy and sexuality, if there are major difficulties between you, we suggest that you address these issues in the relationship before re-evaluating your sexual relationship. Once you are ready to evaluate your sexual relationship (i.e., you feel pretty satisfied with the emotional connection between you, and anger and tension have been satisfactorily addressed), a question that helps start this evaluation is, "Have I ever been involved in any sexual experience that made me feel uncomfortable?" That is a very helpful question for each of you to ask each other as well.

How Do You Rate?

This chapter has provided you with some ways to evaluate your relationship. Now that you have an understanding of what the key ingredients of a relationship are, you can examine how they apply to you as a couple. The following activities are designed to help you assess the status of your relationship and how it has been affected by cancer. See the workbook (*Couples' Corner*) at the end of this book for more structured exercises.

❥ If there were one thing about your relationship you would like to change, what would it be? What can you do to help create that change?

❥ Rate your relationship on a scale of 1 to 10 (10 = highest) on the four important aspects of a couple's relationship. Discuss what you need to do in each area to raise your score.
  • Commitment
  • Connection (through a balance of attachment and independence)
  • Communication
  • Sexual intimacy

❥ Discuss how cancer affects your relationship in the following ways:
  • Does one of you deal with difficult feelings by distancing yourself emotionally or physically from the person who needs you?
  • Does one of you tend to minimize a threat, act overly cheerful all the time, or refuse to acknowledge there's a problem?
  • Are you resentful that your needs are being pushed under the rug because of the illness?
  • Do you tend to blame one another when something terrible happens?
  • Does one of you seem unrealistically optimistic or pessimistic in ways that cause conflict and distance?
  • Do you feel that you or your partner's level of anxiety or emotionality is hurting your relationship?
  • Was your relationship or family life troubled before the diagnosis, and did it get worse afterwards?
  • Is the illness so much on your minds that there's just nothing else you can talk about anymore?
  • Do you have difficulty talking to and listening to one another?
  • Do you feel that cancer has trapped you in a relationship that you wish to escape?

Chapter Four

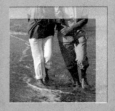

What It Takes
to Create a Good Relationship

It is tempting to focus only on overcoming problems that have come up in a relationship. However, identifying, and then building on, the strengths in a relationship is equally important. Most relationships have good and bad aspects, and any steps a couple can take to enhance the good and minimize the bad are positive. Although it is not realistic to expect a perfect relationship, you can work towards a relationship that is happy and healthy overall.

In this chapter, we will describe characteristics of a healthy relationship —one in which there is ongoing growth, more good times than bad, and an overall sense of satisfaction and security. If you can understand what makes a relationship tick, you will be in a better position to work on your own.

How a Strong, Happy Relationship Looks and Feels

In their book, *The Good Marriage: How & Why Love Lasts*, Judith Wallerstein, Ph.D., and Sandra Blakeslee write about couples with happy and lasting marriages. Dr. Wallerstein interviewed fifty couples who described their marriages as contented and mutually satisfying. These couples were in their first or second marriage, and had been together for at least nine years. Couples were interviewed in the beginning of the study and then again two years later. Based on this research, Wallerstein and Blakeslee describe nine major elements of a good marriage. In the sections below, we'll describe these elements and how they may apply to couples who are facing cancer.

Committed from the Start

We mentioned in Chapter 3 that people who have separated themselves from previous attachments and can devote all of their energy to the current relationship are more likely to have a satisfying relationship. Indeed, Wallerstein and Blakeslee found that each partner in a happy and lasting relationship had successfully separated from the family in which he or she was raised. Their primary love and loyalty became focused on their new family. They were able to rearrange and redefine their relationships with family members from their childhood in order to be fully invested in their marriages. With this steady commitment to each other comes a feeling of comfort and security. Members of the satisfied couples described feeling as though they *always* knew their partner. They see themselves as whole or content, and as worthy of being cherished in the eyes of the partner. Ultimately, partners in satisfying relationships may grow to feel interdependent, as though they could not live without each other.

When a couple confronts cancer, their self-contained unit often expands to include other people. Parents and in-laws, friends, siblings, and others usually rally to their support. This is necessary and can be very helpful. However, as the couple begins to rely on others for things they otherwise would have taken care of between themselves, their sense of unity can suffer at times. For instance, if you discussed important matters with your partner before the cancer, you may now find yourself turning more often to other members of your support network. There may even be times when you purposely refrain from sharing certain information with your partner. Situations like these can undermine the sense of solidarity that is usually a part of any strong marriage.

Separate and Together

Both independence and closeness are important to resilient, happy relationships. Each member of the couple develops a strong sense of who he or she is as a person, as well as an intimate understanding of his or her partner. The knowledge each partner develops about the other's feelings, desires, and life histories helps to strengthen the relationship, creating even greater closeness. Developing such closeness requires that both partners be comfortable expressing their true feelings to each other.

Partners in good relationships have usually learned how to make each other happy. They make efforts to embrace and support each other's interests, even when they may at times prefer to be doing something else. These efforts might involve, for example, going with a partner to a sporting event or joining in the planning and giving of a dinner party. Making such efforts shows the love that each partner feels for the other. The more often these caring behaviors occur, the greater the positive impact they can have on the relationship.

When a couple is dealing with cancer, it may often happen that neither partner feels able to muster the time or energy to do things simply to please the other. Making such symbolic efforts at intimacy may seem like an impossible dream when your attention is directed to more pressing concerns such as sleep, transportation, or control of pain and nausea. It is unlikely to be harmful to your relationship if these intimate moments are put aside at times, such as during the most intensive phase of a highly disruptive treatment. After all, you can also express love for your partner by helping to take care of his or her basic needs. However, building the small kindnesses back into the day-to-day relationship will be important whenever this becomes possible.

The Balancing Act

Having children adds a whole other dimension to a relationship. People in happy, long-term relationships tend to embrace parenthood, while still finding time to spend together privately as a couple. They recognize that there are times when the children's needs take priority, and other times when the marriage must be the first concern. Partners in stable and satisfying relationships are generally able to balance these competing demands.

When illness becomes part of the picture, it can be even more difficult to balance priorities. Some couples may invest much of their time and resources in their relationship, to the exclusion of their children. They may understandably become so focused on the demands of the disease that they inadvertently fail to consider some of their children's needs. At these times you'll need to remember that cancer affects the entire family. Finding a way to talk to your children about the circumstances, and how the illness is likely to impact the family, is an important part of coping as a family (see Chapter 7 for more information). Research suggests that talking about cancer really does help to lower children's anxiety and to improve family communication in general.

On the other hand, some couples may concentrate exclusively on their children's needs in order to avoid dealing with problems in their relationship. Directing all of your energy to your children can indeed be a way to distract yourself from other—perhaps more painful—issues. However, if this goes on for an extended period and problems in your relationship remain neglected, it can ultimately lead to an unsatisfying relationship that may become strikingly apparent after the children have grown and moved out. The take-home message is that there are times when your children's needs take the front seat, but not to let lengthy periods go by without addressing your needs as a couple.

In Sickness and in Health

Couples in enduring relationships maintain their commitment even through hard times. By doing so, they can overcome crises, such as a diagnosis of cancer. Any crisis requires change and adjustment. When severe stress assaults a relationship, it affects both partners. It can also set off a chain reaction of responses and events that affect other people in the family. All of a sudden you may find yourself facing questions that you never had to face before, like, "Is my partner going to be alive in two years?" Often the answers to these questions imply new roles for each partner.

Partners in an optimal relationship make every effort to share the burden of a crisis without giving in to the temptation to find someone to blame. They also are able to separate out the crisis from other areas of their life. By doing so, satisfied couples can keep the "big picture" in focus. In the middle of the crisis, they often make efforts to do something enjoyable that provides distraction and relief from the situation. The couples in Dr. Wallerstein's study worked at trying to keep destructive feelings and actions out of their marriage during crisis. They often took steps in advance to make sure that a crisis from the outside did not provoke a crisis within the relationship.

When one person in a relationship becomes ill, it is especially important to keep the channels of communication open, talk about feelings, and accommodate each other. Neglecting these aspects of an intimate relationship can have negative consequences. For example, the healthy partner may offer basic caregiving in a way that seems forced and lacks emotional warmth. This may be the style of dealing with illness that the healthy partner learned while growing up, based on the assumption that sick people like to go off alone to heal without any fuss (see pages 16–19). If this type of caregiving is not what the sick person wants, he or she may feel disappointed and may even feel that the situation is intolerable. Such missteps can be very damaging to a relationship, but they can be easily avoided by openly expressing your needs and desires. This is usually a much safer bet than assuming that your partner is a mind reader.

Open Communication

Couples in happy, long-lasting relationships build an environment that allows for free expression of differences, anger, and disappointment. This means that a person can get angry and still count on his or her partner to be there after the anger goes away. Both partners understand that it is better to tell each other exactly how they feel than to let small annoyances build into big issues.

During the course of an illness, it is normal for people to feel anger, even though people often berate themselves for getting angry during their partner's illness. Expressing such feelings in a constructive, direct way can be beneficial, and efforts to quash strong feelings of anger can cause damage to the relationship (see Chapter 5). Even though it can be difficult to address issues when they first arise, especially during an experience with cancer, try to share with your partner how you are feeling as soon as the problem develops. It is easy to convince yourself that an issue is too small to bother your partner or that it is something you'll eventually get used to. However, if you don't address your concerns up front, they tend to build over time.

Believe it or not, arguing "well"—in a constructive way—can actually be a source of satisfaction in relationships. Anger can be expressed within the relationship without hurting each other, airing dirty laundry, or name-calling. It can ultimately be healing. Expressing anger constructively is a way to deal honestly with your partner and can build intimacy. This requires a willingness to face not only your fears, but to share them also. In Chapter 9, we explain how couples can build more emotional intimacy.

Couples can lower the heat in an argument by using a well-placed humorous comment, or just taking a break from the discussion. This can take the potential of destructiveness out of anger. One effective way of dealing with anger is simply to ask for what you want from your partner instead of fighting. For people who take pride in being self-sufficient, this can be difficult, but it's worth the effort.

Some people find it helpful to pull themselves out of the heat of the moment, acting as if they feel "curious" about the argument rather than mad or fearful. This more neutral stance can help to put an argument into perspective and make it less painful and upsetting. For example, asking questions like, "Gee, I wonder why I am reacting so strongly to this?" or, "Boy, he really seems upset. I wonder what is really behind this emotion?" can help a person to understand the situation in a constructive way without allowing strong emotions to get in the way. This objectivity can help partners devise creative solutions to the problems they face.

Another uncomfortable emotion that may arise is a feeling of being disconnected from your partner. Do not worry if this happens occasionally. Commitment is an important "rudder" that helps couples ride out the waves of arguments or periods of feeling distant from one another. Despite feeling angry or disconnected occasionally, many couples come to an understanding that *no matter what*, they can see it through together. One happily married woman jokingly said, "I figured if my husband ever actually murdered someone, I would call it off. Anything short of that was negotiable."

Mature and committed couples usually believe that even when they do disagree or feel separate or distant, they can wait it out and eventually things will get resolved (or, if not resolved, will diminish in importance). Whatever the issue is, they have confidence that they will eventually get through it or past it. These couples value their commitment over most external and internal forces that conspire to separate them. They refuse to give up on their partnership, and their shared history of many years drives their continued commitment. This was certainly the case with Yvonne and Bob (described in the Introduction). They had both been previously married and understood the kind of commitment it takes to make a relationship work. Their relationship became closer as they shared their feelings about Bob's cancer, and they found strength in each other.

The unshakable commitment of satisfied couples may be a symptom rather than a cause of their relationship satisfaction. For example, partners who are particularly well matched may have a stronger commitment to one another because of what the relationship offers them. Also, remember that we are describing the experience of people in optimal relationships. We realize that some readers may feel more "stuck" in their difficulties than the couples we're describing in this chapter. We address such challenges and solutions in Sections 2 and 3.

Happiness Behind Closed Doors

A common aspect of most long-lasting relationships is a rich and pleasurable sexual relationship. A couple's sex life can help them feel close even if there are some issues they have been unable to resolve through discussion. Establishing a satisfying sex life requires mutual trust. The reward is a closer relationship.

In a partnership, sex should be balanced. Both partners should be able to give and receive pleasure. There are some common problems that may disrupt this balance. Men often note that over time, their partners do not seem to have the same interest, energy, focus, or passion for sex. If they believe that their partner is just going along with sex to be agreeable, sex may become less enjoyable for them. Women, on the other hand, often wish men would slow down and take pleasure in the process of having sex, without exclusively focusing on the goal of reaching orgasm.

As a relationship matures, attentiveness may replace the passion that drove sexual activity during the honeymoon phase of the relationship. Part of being attentive to your sexual relationship is talking about it together. Talk about what you enjoy in lovemaking. You don't have to provide your partner with a long description or a detailed guide. You can simply compliment him or her on something that made you feel especially tender, aroused, or loved. It may be less comfortable to talk to your partner during the actual sexual encounter. If that is true, you may find that you can say something before or after making love that highlights the experience or that sets the stage for your next encounter. This may be as simple as saying that you feel especially close to your partner after making love. Often, intimate partners do not share these simple, but important, thoughts and feelings with one another.

One rule in relationships, especially sexual ones, is that if you make an effort to enjoy yourself, chances are your partner will be pleased too. Half of the fun of having sex is bringing pleasure to the other person. When you are expressing your pleasure, your partner is happy to take some responsibility for bringing that pleasure to you. We talk about how to maintain and strengthen your sexual relationship—even in the face of cancer—in Chapter 10.

Laughter Is the Best Medicine

Happy love relationships involve humor. Boredom is avoided by sharing fun, interests, and friends. The ways in which a husband and wife banter or tease each other can be very intimate and can develop into a shared secret language.

Even during the cancer experience, couples may find moments where the absurdity and strangeness of it all can cause them to collapse in laughter. Those moments may be rare, but are precious to couples. Some couples have an easy time finding humor in difficult situations, since it is their habit anyway. For example, when Yvonne walked into Bob's hospital room during one stay, his first comment was, "I'm exhausted—I just finished my exercises." Yvonne was puzzled since Bob could not easily get out of bed. It turned out that Bob was referring to his morning aerobic exercises with "Daisy," an attractive and vivacious woman whose show he had watched several times on TV. As Yvonne learned to her delight and amusement, his "exercises" consisted of moving his eyes back and forth during Daisy's vigorous movements on the screen.

Some of the awful and awkward moments that patients find themselves in when dealing with cancer can be shared only with the people closest to you. For example, when asked a question that he didn't feel like answering, one patient who was diagnosed with brain cancer had a habit of replying, "Don't ask me—I have a brain tumor!" He would say this with an ironic smile. Although his situation was not fun or amusing, he found humor in the experience when he could. Sharing humor with someone who can appreciate it is invaluable.

Friends Who Care

Partners in satisfying relationships offer each other nurturance and comfort, continuous encouragement, and support. This support is based on genuine compassion and an intimate understanding of the other person's needs.

Although cancer requires some adjustments, couples can learn how to take care of each other, often with small gestures. Fred brings Bonnie coffee in bed each morning, since he knows she has a tough time getting out of bed. Yvonne calls Bob in the middle of the day with a tidbit of news or a thought, simply because it pleases them both. A strong, caring relationship can provide the cancer patient with a sense of security, a feeling that someone will be there, regardless of what adversity may arise.

Rekindling the Flame

Couples in long-lasting relationships often find ways to keep alive the romantic love that their relationship began with. At the same time, they are able to accept the changes in each other and the relationship over time. The relationship is built on shared memories and history, but it also evolves to accommodate the realities of the present.

After the honeymoon phase, partners can come to see each other without distortion, valuing each other as much as they value themselves. They give without expecting anything in return, freely exchanging love between them. During this stage of a relationship, some people may describe their partners as passionate friends. This type of relationship is transforming, meaning that it actually provides the nourishment that allows each partner to grow and change as a person.

In the process of keeping their relationship strong over time, partners share their hopes and dreams with one another and build a shared sense of meaning together. The process of finding meaning and purpose in everyday experiences happens naturally when both partners feel unconditionally accepted and loved.

It can also happen that a relationship that was previously stuck in a stalemate can unexpectedly shift into a period of renewed growth. Couples who are able to transform unsatisfying relationships into satisfying ones typically have a lot invested in their relationships to begin with. They do not take divorce lightly, so they are motivated to look for other options. Even though it can be painful, sometimes the fading of one aspect of a relationship creates room for other areas to grow. For example, sometimes a transformation such as this may happen when one partner has stopped unrealistically longing to be rescued from personal problems by the other. After shedding the old skin of the unsatisfying dependency, the previously dependent partner grows in self-reliance. This can allow both partners to discover more satisfying roles.

Transformations may also happen when an external stress leads to a crisis for one or both partners. For Yvonne and Bob, the crisis of cancer sparked a kind of growth in the relationship. It was almost as though Bob's life-threatening illness sped up time for both of them. When both partners, and the relationship, enter into such a period of growth, there is often a renewed connection. It may feel like falling in love again.

Principles in Action

Richard and Rachel have been married for forty-three years. They have two grown children, both in their late thirties. They (and their friends) would say they have a "good marriage." But it hasn't always felt that way. Three years ago, Rachel found a lump in her breast.

THEY MET WHEN BOTH WERE IN GRADUATE SCHOOL, and they were attracted to each other instantly. (That attraction has never gone completely away, although they joke about the times when the feeling of attraction and love was on a "long vacation.") After a yearlong courtship, during which they had many intimate talks and loving moments, Richard and Rachel married. They were idealistic about the world and about each other. They settled in a community where they could live out their dreams of helping others. They were dedicated to serving the poor and uneducated in the rural southern county where they lived. Both shared a passion for working on behalf of the civil rights movement in the 1960s. These were exciting years, but often stressful. The work Richard and Rachel chose did not pay well. While much of the work was rewarding, some of it was frustrating.

Over time, they began to see things in each other that were less than appealing. For Richard, he had never realized how frugal and concerned about money Rachel was. He knew that they didn't have much, but he felt like he had to ask permission to spend any money. Every now and then, he wanted to go out to dinner and just forget about their responsibilities, but Rachel simply couldn't see doing that in their current circumstances. From Rachel's perspective, it seemed Richard was more focused on the materialistic side of life than she had ever dreamed. He harped about getting new furniture and going out to expensive dinners. To her, those things seemed secondary to their life's work.

Soon, they became parents. Rachel decided that she really wanted to stay home and take care of the children, just as her mother had done with her. Richard agreed to the arrangement. Their personality differences were highlighted by their different parenting styles. Rachel's parents thought that if you "spared the rod, you spoiled the child." While she didn't spank the children often, she was the disciplinarian of the family. Richard was the "fun daddy" when he came home in the evening. He seemed to avoid setting limits on the kids. Although Rachel appreciated that he was fun and jovial with the children, she got tired of her role as the firm parent. She and Richard had many arguments about parenting styles over the years.

After a few incidents when they openly disagreed about parenting in front of their children, Richard and Rachel made a pact to present a united front to them in the future. For the most part, they kept their pact.

As the children grew and eventually left home, Rachel resumed her career. At this point in her life, she was drawn to working with refugees, many of whom were homeless. Richard began working with a nonprofit corporation that raised funds for elder care. The couple felt their tensions easing, since now they were both doing what they really wanted to do with their lives. Richard had been able to open Rachel up to the idea of spending some money on themselves, and

Rachel had curbed Richard's habit of making impulsive purchases. They accepted their different spending styles, and even came to admire each other's opposing views on money management.

They agreed that they had neglected their marriage while they were actively raising the kids, and they were delighted to learn that they still had things to talk about with each other. They still found each other interesting and still felt there was something new to learn both from and about each other. As Richard explains it, "There's always been that little feeling inside when I think about Rachel or see her. It's just that feeling of love that never totally goes away. There are days I really don't like her very much, but even those are pretty rare these days. Plus if I wait it out, I usually feel differently in a day or two. If I don't, I know the problem is usually something inside me, rather than a problem with Rachel. So, that's what I look at."

Even though they successfully dealt with some major personality differences, Richard and Rachel still had their share of conflict in their marriage. Sometimes their discussions were extremely painful, and both felt lonely and isolated from the other. There were moments for Rachel when she felt Richard made such selfish decisions that she thought about leaving. She was tired of always having to take his agenda into consideration. She found, though, that if she focused on what she needed, it made it much easier to understand that Richard had his own needs as well. With this change in focus, she was able to accept his limitations more easily, as well as her own.

At one point in the relationship, Richard and Rachel each lost a parent. That was a very difficult year. But they were proud of the way they supported each other through it. They didn't always like how the other person expressed grief, but they found that if they talked things out, both of them would usually feel better. There was no question that they were there for each other when times were tough.

Rachel and Richard always had a good sex life. Like all other aspects of their life, it seemed to improve or falter with changing life circumstances. They nurtured each other in many ways. They helped take care of each other, so they felt loving more often than not. Rachel took pride in enclosing little notes in Richard's coat pockets. Sometimes they were just a joke, other times they were tender and serious. Richard was physically affectionate most of the time—holding her hand in public, putting his arm around her protectively. In times like these, the two of them felt like a team.

When Rachel found a lump in her breast, her first concern was her husband's reaction. Although he didn't often say it, he depended on his wife almost completely for his emotional support. In spite of Rachel's worries, Richard rose to the occasion. He accompanied Rachel to the biopsy, which revealed stage II breast cancer. He fielded calls from concerned family and friends, cooked dinners, researched her disease on the Internet, and never left her side during appointments or treatments. Richard and Rachel realized that they were indeed fortunate to have had the life they shared together.

When they thought back on their tough times, and how angry and worked up they could get about things, they simply laughed at themselves. They found it funny how their attitudes had changed since they were naive twenty-somethings who thought that they could save the world. Now they decided they would be happy saving themselves and their marriage. With new appreciation for life's many twists and turns, Richard and Rachel look forward to both the good times and the bad. Their marriage is "good enough" to see them through all of it—even cancer.

To sum up, good relationships are often built when each partner is free to invest all of his or her resources in the relationship from the beginning. Usually, each partner has moved away from previous attachments. Good relationships have a balance of independence and closeness. Children's needs are balanced with the need to invest in the couple's relationship. Commitment is steadfast despite hardship. Each partner feels free to be honest and open, including expression of his or her sexual responses and desires. There is shared humor, and mutual nurturing and support. Good relationships often have a fluid quality, as each partner and the relationship grows and adapts to changing realities over time.

SECTION 2
Challenges

Couples typically face many challenges in their confrontation with cancer. It often presents couples with difficult new issues. It can also make existing problems worse. By understanding the specific ways that people react to such challenges, you can be prepared to navigate the course.

In this section, we will explore many of the ways that cancer can affect individuals and their relationships. We will discuss how relationships can be influenced by the intense emotional reactions that can arise with cancer, such as anger and depression. We also discuss some unique problems that couples may have struggled with even before cancer was diagnosed, such as persistent conflicts, alcoholism, or domestic abuse. Finally, we'll discuss how cancer can interact with other specific aspects of a couple's lifestyle, such as their careers and parenting roles.

Chapter Five

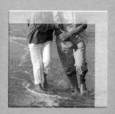

Emotions,
Relationships, and Cancer

S trong emotions are natural and common during an experience with cancer. In this chapter, we discuss how these emotional reactions can affect your relationship. We will focus on two of the most difficult emotional experiences—depression and anger—that can be overwhelming when they become intense or persist for a long time. We'll also examine different styles of coping with emotions and how these differences can affect couple relationships. Last but not least, we'll look at the physical and emotional aspects of sexual intimacy.

Depression Affects Relationships

One or both partners may develop depression at any time in the course of a relationship. The stress of a cancer diagnosis increases the risk of becoming depressed for both partners. When one partner does become depressed, it can have a harmful effect on the quality of life for both partners.

Without treatment, some people go through a negative cycle in which depression affects relationship satisfaction; decreased relationship satisfaction, in turn, worsens the depression. Problems in a relationship can also increase the likelihood of getting depressed in the first place. The flip side of this is that a satisfying relationship can help protect people from becoming depressed or help relieve depression when it occurs. Research has shown that women who have close, affectionate relationships with their spouses are less likely to be depressed than those who do not.

Depression affects both the depressed person and his or her partner. Living with a person who is depressed can be stressful, just as it is stressful to go through depression yourself. In one study, almost half of the spouses of depressed partners reported distress that was serious enough to warrant psychiatric consultation. This highlights the importance of paying attention to the emotional well-being of all members of your family when one person is depressed.

Caregivers often report that depression was the most difficult issue that they dealt with during their partner's illness. Even under the best of circumstances, it is hard to watch a partner experience the feelings that accompany depression, such as pain, hopelessness, and anguish. It can also be difficult to know how to handle these feelings when they are expressed. One positive step that the partner of a depressed patient can take is to let the health care team know about any changes in the patient's mood and behavior that may signal depression.

Depression: What It's All About

The stress of dealing with an illness like cancer can cause many people to feel sad or hopeless. Sometimes they are able to get over "the blues" in a short time. Sometimes, however, these feelings can persist for a long time, and they may even get stronger over time. When a person feels sad, pessimistic, or hopeless for several weeks or even months, and when these feelings interfere with managing day-to-day affairs, the person may be suffering from depression.

Depression is an emotional state that is more excessive and prolonged than a typical, manageable emotional response to stress. Certain people have a higher risk of developing depression than others. People are not to blame for developing depression, and having depression is not a sign of a character flaw. Factors that increase the risk for depression include losses; physical, social, or emotional stresses; and having a family history of depression or mood disorders.

Depression often creates a downward spiral. When people feel down, they don't have the energy to solve problems. When the problems get worse, they feel worse, and so on. This downward spiral must be interrupted as quickly as possible to prevent a worsening of the depression, so early treatment is necessary. Such treatment may involve emotional support or counseling, as well as antidepressant medications. Some feelings of sadness or anxiety are normal responses to the stresses and uncertainties of chronic illness, so these feelings will not completely go away with treatment. However, treatment can keep these emotional responses within normal bounds so that they are manageable and not crippling.

In addition to feelings of sadness, other symptoms of depression include appetite changes (too much or too little appetite), sleep problems, difficulty concentrating, and a lack of energy or desire to do things. Increased alcohol use may also be a sign of depression. If the person with cancer is depressed, he or she may have problems coping with the illness and the life changes that come with it. Sometimes these coping difficulties become so intense that the depressed person thinks about suicide as a way out. If this becomes the case for you or your partner, be sure to contact your doctor immediately.

In the context of a medical illness, depression may be caused or worsened by physical pain (especially when not treated adequately), medication side effects, or chemical imbalances in the body due to the cancer. When depression occurs for these reasons, changes in medical treatments may help, so let health care providers know about the depression (see Chapter 12).

In the following example, Keith's depression is directly affecting his wife's mood and feelings of optimism.

KEITH EXHIBITS MANY OF THE SYMPTOMS OF DEPRESSION. He is experiencing low motivation, sadness, loss of interest in things, and withdrawal from social contact. These symptoms may have been made worse by the steroid medicines he took throughout his bone marrow transplant. His depression is having a major impact on his family. Alicia is doing tasks Keith would normally be able to take care of, and she is becoming exhausted and resentful. Keith is like a different person, and Alicia misses her former companion and support. There are times when she feels hopeless about their situation, even though medically her husband is doing well and has a good prognosis.

About Depression

What to Look for

❧ People who have symptoms of depression every day, for most of the day, or for at least two weeks may have clinical depression. These symptoms include:
  • Persistent sad or "empty" mood almost every day for most of the day
  • Loss of interest or pleasure in all, or almost all, activities most of the day
  • Eating problems (loss of appetite or overeating), or significant weight loss or gain
  • Sleep disturbances (insomnia, early waking, or oversleeping)
  • Noticeable restlessness almost every day
  • Decreased energy, or fatigue almost every day
  • Feelings of guilt, worthlessness, or helplessness
  • Difficulty concentrating, remembering, or making decisions
  • Thoughts of death or suicide, or attempts at suicide

❧ If you or your partner have any of these symptoms, you should talk with your health care provider about depression and the possible ways to treat it.

The Benefits of Treatment

❧ It can reduce pain and suffering.

❧ It can relieve the symptoms of depression.

❧ It can help most people feel better and return to daily activities within several weeks.

❧ The earlier you get treatment, the sooner you can begin to feel better.

Other Things to Do

❧ In addition to seeking professional treatment, there are several other steps that may help to decrease the severity of the symptoms of depression (although these are not intended as a substitute for professional help):
  • Schedule activities that are pleasant, comforting, or give you a feeling of accomplishment.
  • Increase the amount of contact you have with other people.
  • Use a problem-solving approach to tackle some of the day-to-day problems that are contributing to your feelings of depression.
  • Join a support group.

Anger

In any relationship, it is natural to feel angry at times. Feelings of anger can range from a mild irritation to an intense rage. Talking about anger in constructive ways can be a positive step that sets the stage for healing and calm to be restored to the relationship. Venting anger isn't always positive, however. Anger that is expressed as an attack on another person can be destructive. Harmful expressions of anger are more likely when the angry feelings are intense.

Sometimes, intense anger can occur when people allow small issues to build up over time instead of dealing with them when the emotions are not as strong and are more easily manageable. Intense emotions can also arise when a situation reopens wounds from earlier in the relationship or from childhood. Regardless of the source of the anger, you can often make strides towards a positive outcome if you are able to express the feelings of disappointment, fear, hurt, or frustration that are behind the anger, rather than attacking your partner for causing those feelings.

Sometimes couples argue about who is at fault in an argument, rather than working towards a solution to the disagreement. In the heat of anger, people tend to exaggerate their side of the story, using provocative words like "you always" or "you never." This kind of "attack" language almost always causes the other person to become defensive, and greatly lowers the chance that anything positive will come of the discussion.

Having cancer can create feelings of anger that have no rational target. You may feel outraged that your career has been derailed or that your partner can no longer continue to work part time. When you have such strong feelings about a major life change, the slightest provocation can cause intense irritation. Some people may express anger when they are uncomfortable talking about other feelings, such as anxiety or sadness. Anger and depression can go together, and each one tends to make the other more intense.

Styles of Conflict

One of the most common complaints of couples in therapy is that they have problems resolving conflicts. This often happens because the partners have different styles of dealing with conflict, which they may have learned earlier in life. When these styles do not mesh well, it can be the source of a great deal of frustration in a relationship. In the sections below, we'll look at some common styles of dealing with conflict. (We discuss ways to resolve conflicts in Chapter 8.)

The Cold Shoulder Approach

Some people use silence and withdrawal rather than words to express anger. They may go to great pains to avoid talking about problems. People who are generally uncomfortable with being close and expressing feelings (see Chapter 2) may be more likely to withdraw during a conflict. They may fear that their emotions are so intense that they can't be expressed without causing serious harm to the relationship. If your partner has this style, you are more likely to get a better response from him or her if you raise the issue when emotions have cooled down a bit.

The Catharsis Approach

Some people are at the opposite extreme from those who use the cold shoulder to deal with conflict—they let their partners know what is on their minds without considering the consequences. People who deal with conflict in this way may yell, shout, or even throw things (see Chapter 6 for more information on domestic violence). They may say things in the heat of anger that are hard to forgive or forget, leaving the recipient of the harsh language feeling bruised and battered. Fortunately, people with this style often are also very expressive of their love and positive feelings towards their partners, and this can go a long way towards healing any damage caused. Still, it is better to avoid causing the damage in the first place.

There are some particularly harmful actions that people who have a tendency to "let it all out" should do their best to avoid. In general, these include anything that leaves the partner feeling belittled, ashamed, or afraid. Some examples include: discounting your partner's ideas or needs; putting your partner down by making a joke; accusing and blaming; judging and criticizing; threatening; and name-calling. One of the best ways to avoid giving such harmful messages is to discuss problems using what are called "I" statements. These kinds of statements are phrased in such a way that they convey the impact your partner's behavior has on you, rather than labeling your partner. For example, it is much more helpful to say, "*I* really get angry when you ignore me" than, "*You* are such a jerk."

IN THE BEGINNING OF BONNIE AND FRED'S MARRIAGE, she was stunned by his thoughtless outbursts. He tended to hold onto issues from the past and pull them out in the middle of an argument. After a while, Bonnie confronted Fred about how this behavior hurt her. They worked on ways to argue more appropriately, with less finger-pointing and hysteria. With practice, Fred was able to change these bad habits because he was highly motivated to avoid hurting Bonnie or their relationship.

The Escape Approach

Some people's method of choice for dealing with conflict is to escape the situation. This can be done in various ways. People may drink alcohol or take drugs, go on long, expensive shopping trips, or work constantly. In the extreme, somebody that uses this strategy may leave the house and not return for days. The partner left at home is often frantically worried, and then relieved when the person returns. Because his or her worry has been relieved in the short term, the problem that led to this behavior is often ignored, even though the conflict is not resolved. Escape is another method of dealing with conflict that is often used by "withdrawers" (people who are uncomfortable with emotional closeness). In such cases, the partner who wants to be close (the "pursuer") may be so afraid of abandonment that he or she is willing to give in to whatever his or her partner wants.

Power Struggles

Sometimes conflicts in a relationship become a way of competing for power or dominance. When this is the case, both partners wind up feeling controlled and not understood by each other. This is the time to listen to and respect your partner's position. Avoid manipulative statements such as, "If you loved me, you would _____." These kinds of statements may signal a lack of respect for the other person's feelings and desires. Although sacrificing some of your wishes to please your partner can be a way to show your love, such sacrifices should not always be one sided, and they should be made in an atmosphere of mutual respect.

Couples often have power struggles regarding space, money, having children, and other lifestyle issues. To complicate matters, sometimes these clashes may reflect deeper differences in personal values or beliefs. It is worth exploring these differences by expressing what these issues mean to you and asking your partner to talk about what they mean to him or her. Once you better understand each other's needs and where they come from, it is helpful for each of you to think of possible solutions that are acceptable to you and yet meet your partner's needs as much as possible.

It is not essential to come to a compromise to resolve a disagreement. How you discuss these differences with your partner can be more important than actually resolving them. There may be some issues that touch on your core value system, and you may be unwilling to compromise on these issues because they are central to who you are. One such core value is that of religious preferences. For example, a woman who has been happily married for twenty-seven years, states, "I attend a Methodist church, and my husband attends a Catholic church. I wish we could attend together, but the differences are just too great for either of us to feel comfortable in each other's churches. So, we lose the togetherness, but individually we are spiritually satisfied." It is often a healthy solution to agree to disagree on certain things, rather than allowing yourself to be frustrated by trying to persuade your partner to give in to your wishes.

Problems with Showing Emotions

Having a partner who openly expresses his or her emotions can be very comforting. People who are good at expressing warmth make it clear that they plan to stick with their partners even if tough times occur. They are able to respond in a caring way when their partners express emotions like fear or sadness. Unfortunately, some people have great difficulty expressing and responding to emotions. If two partners have mismatched styles, it can be frustrating and difficult, especially during the stress of an experience with cancer. You already know that cancer triggers strong feelings. If your partner comes across as emotionally distant or unresponsive, it can add to the difficulty of coping with these feelings.

JANE AND MARK HAVE BEEN MARRIED FOR OVER TEN YEARS. Mark cares deeply for Jane, but he has a hard time showing it. He grew up in a home where he was taught to "keep a stiff upper lip," and no one in his family was comfortable giving hugs or saying, "I love you" aloud. So Mark shows that he cares for Jane by doing, rather than by saying. He thinks that Jane should know how much he loves her by all the things that he does for her and their household, such as fixing the car and mowing the lawn.

Jane was recently diagnosed with cervical cancer, and this has put a serious strain on their relationship. Mark has been diligent in helping take her to appointments and pitching in with the housecleaning. However, every time Jane tries to talk about how she is feeling about the situation, Mark is unresponsive. He isn't able to express his reactions to her illness or how it is affecting him and their relationship. All he says is "Everything will be fine."

If you want a close relationship and you are involved with someone who doesn't freely express his or her emotions, you may feel as if you are doing all of the work in the relationship, while your own needs are not getting met. In contrast, your partner may be expending more energy trying to maintain a safe distance from you than trying to be close.

There are a lot of reasons why some people may be uncomfortable expressing tender feelings. In the scene above, Mark had difficulty because he simply was not used to expressing himself this way, having had no prior experience with this kind of self-expression during his upbringing. Some people may withdraw from closeness because they are anxious about committing to a long-term relationship. Others who were adored and catered to early in life may have difficulty focusing on someone else's needs as adults. Some people may be distracted by worries or be so analytical that they get bogged down in thoughts and have a hard time being spontaneous. There are also people who are overly concerned about looking foolish or risking rejection, so they keep their conversations at a superficial level in order to avoid these risks.

Intimacy and Sexual Concerns

Intimacy is a broad term that encompasses many areas, including affection, expressiveness, compatibility, and sexuality. In a nutshell, people who are intimate are comfortable being themselves when they are together. An intimate relationship is a loyal partnership, characterized by feeling closer to your partner than to anyone else. An intimate relationship is one in which you can share your innermost thoughts and feelings and still be accepted and loved. All of the previously described problems in this chapter—depression, anger, and difficulty showing emotions—can decrease the level of intimacy in a relationship.

While your level of intimacy with your partner may grow throughout your relationship, passion is likely to ebb and flow over time. Both intimacy and passion contribute to our enjoyment of sex. Sexuality involves being in touch with the passionate, playful, adventurous side of yourself, but sex is more meaningful if intimacy and expressiveness are high. It is possible to have good sex without having a good relationship, and vice versa. However, good sex is much more likely to happen in a relationship that involves commitment, intimacy, and passion.

What Is "Good Sex?"

A reasonable goal for good sex is that it is tension reducing and satisfies each person's needs and wishes at least some of the time. Appreciation and acceptance of your partner enhances good sex. In a good marriage, sex and love are usually intertwined.

Sex and Cancer

When one member of a couple is diagnosed with cancer, his or her first concern is survival. As soon as treatment begins, however, there may be other concerns. For example, even if treatment goes well, patients wonder how normal their lives can be, including sex. People often don't talk about the effects of cancer treatment on sexuality. Yet, sex is usually more satisfying if you can openly discuss it with your partner, and this is especially important when one partner has cancer.

Being as specific as possible about your sexual preferences and needs helps your partner meet those needs. Couples must also discuss "sex logistics"— the where, how, and when aspects of their sexual relationship. Cancer can affect sex logistics in a number of ways. A woman being treated with chemotherapy for cancer may not be able to have sex when her white blood cell count is very low. A man who just had prostate surgery may not be able to ejaculate in the same way he did before surgery. Cancer treatments like radiation therapy or chemotherapy can also cause fatigue, which may decrease the desire for sex.

Most people have needs for physical closeness that do not involve sex. The need to be touched, caressed, kissed, and hugged is universal. Most of us want to feel welcome in our partner's space and want to be physically welcomed when we encounter our partner. Expressing warmth when in each other's presence is a part of intimacy.

Physical intimacy is particularly important when a person's body image has changed because of cancer. Scars, amputation, weight loss or gain, hair loss, and ostomies are all significant changes that may be difficult for couples to adapt to. It is important to pay close attention to the feelings of the partner with cancer for how to deal with these changes. Often it is helpful to wait until the patient feels comfortable discussing his or her feelings about the change before progressing to touching and gradually returning to sexual intimacy. It is crucial for the healthy partner to acknowledge the loss that the partner with cancer feels, but also to assure him or her that your love is unchanged.

Some people are especially likely to be distressed by sexual problems. Younger cancer patients tend to be more emotionally upset about sexual problems than older patients. Being unmarried can increase the level of distress that people experience in response to sexual problems, as single men and women may have less confidence that their partners will continue to love them in spite of a sexual problem. Similarly, new couples are more affected by sexual concerns than those who have been together for years. Finally, people with a history of sexual trauma or previous sexual problems are more likely to be troubled by the sexual impact of cancer.

The first year after cancer treatment is the most common time for sexual problems to emerge. Loss of sexual desire is one of the most common complaints from both men and women. This change in desire can result from depression, feelings of unattractiveness, the use of certain medications, and physical discomfort or ill health. Fear of pain during intercourse or anxiety about erections can also interfere with your sexual life. Adjusting to these changes can be difficult. Learning what can be done to relieve these problems, talking openly with your partner, and finding new ways of expressing love and intimacy can all be reassuring. In Chapter 10, we will explore in details ways you and your partner can create, maintain, or strengthen your sexual life while coping with cancer.

Infertility

Infertility may be an issue for survivors of childhood cancer as well as for adults who have undergone certain types of cancer treatment. Although infertility is a physical problem, it can have psychological effects. Men or women who are unable to conceive a child may feel defective or incomplete. Some people may have a difficult time understanding such feelings, believing that the person should simply be happy to be alive instead of being upset about the inability to conceive a child. But people can be devastated to find out that they cannot have children, which may affect their sense of worth as well as their relationship.

Giving up the idea of having one's biological child is a profound loss for many cancer survivors and their partners. Infertility serves as a blow to a person's self-esteem and may also feed into an irrational guilt about having cancer. If one of the partners seems to be the responsible party for the infertility, there is often guilt and self-blame.

Infertility often brings up intense emotions of anger, sadness, and loss. The emotional turmoil and stress that come with infertility can have several negative effects. Within the relationship, conflict and tension may increase, and one or both partners may become emotionally withdrawn. Sometimes the infertile person even fears that the condition will cause the relationship to end. Infertility can also affect a couple's outside relationships. Some couples are uncomfortable discussing infertility or infertility treatment even with close friends and family, and this may lead them to withdraw from social situations.

Even when infertility can be treated successfully, the current treatments are usually extremely costly. Adoption, often presented as the best solution to infertility, can be expensive and has many potential pros and cons. Adoptions may be complicated by cancer, as agencies may need to investigate the status of the cancer before agreeing to an adoption. Regardless of how a couple ultimately chooses to deal with infertility, the process often involves many hard choices. Consulting with professionals who can help with the emotional and physical aspects of infertility can help you and your partner successfully negotiate infertility. In Chapter 11, we will explain how cancer treatment may affect fertility and how fertility may be protected or treated in some cases.

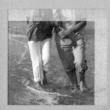

Chapter Six

Couples
in Conflict

Over the course of a relationship, it is natural for a couple to face many problems and crises—some worse than others. So when a couple is faced with the additional stresses of cancer, these difficulties are magnified. In this chapter, we discuss several problems that can have major effects on relationships—recurrent (or core) arguments, extramarital affairs, divorce, domestic violence, and the abuse of alcohol or other drugs. When a couple is confronted with any of these situations, their relationship comes to a crossroad. Unless they take the necessary actions to remedy these situations, serious and permanent damage to the relationship can result.

Core Arguments

Many couples argue about the same issues over and over again. Often, despite hours of discussion, the underlying differences remain unresolved. Even though couples may experience dramatic changes in themselves and their circumstances over the years, they often continue to argue about variations on the same themes. Such arguments are known as core arguments. Here are some examples:

- Ted believes in a debt-free life. His wife, Rebecca, believes some debt is acceptable. She would like to borrow some money to spend on home improvements, but Ted rejects the idea.

- Judy wants to have children. Sam does not.

- Ron hates housework and feels that he works hard enough at his job that he shouldn't have to work at home. Even though Wendy works part-time, she would still like Ron to share in the responsibilities of running their household.

- Eric believes in giving kids unconditional love and letting them make their own mistakes. Karen feels it is important that kids have structure and discipline.

- Sara has cancer, and her oncologist feels that her prognosis for long-term survival is not good. Chris is an optimist and wants to focus on beating the cancer. Sara finds Chris's continuously hopeful attitude difficult to take because she really needs to talk about the worst-case scenario. Chris chides her for being negative whenever she introduces the topic.

When couples are faced with fundamental differences in such important matters, they must learn to cope with their differences, or they will remain frustrated by them. If couples do not successfully resolve core arguments, their relationship can become gridlocked. Each partner may simply refuse to budge from their position, leaving no room for progress. This lack of progress may leave each person feeling frustrated, hurt, or rejected. Eventually, the partners may begin to disengage from the relationship to avoid these uncomfortable emotions. Although this disengagement may bring some short-term relief, it does so at the expense of potentially causing serious harm to the relationship. Even the drastic step of ending a relationship may only be a short-term solution, because in many cases, the same issues resurface in the next relationship.

Core arguments can have such powerful effects because basic values are often at stake. Sometimes these values are so basic to us that they define who we are. When facing something that appears to be a core argument, be aware of your values and the extent to which you are willing to compromise these values in consideration for your partner's values. Some values are so important to us that we are unwilling to compromise on them at all. You can respect

Gridlock

Your relationship may be gridlocked in a core argument if:
- You feel personally rejected by your partner because of the argument.

- You talk and talk and feel that you get nowhere.

- You are inflexible in your position and so is your partner.

- You have unusually intense feelings of hurt or anger when you discuss certain topics.

- You seem to have lost the ability to laugh together or show affection for each other.

- The arguments seem to become more personal over time.

- You have argued so much and so fruitlessly over and over again that you have given up and withdrawn from each other.

your partner's values even if you do not share them. If such values are not respected, it can cause serious problems in the relationship.

Partners do not necessarily have to agree on the same position when resolving core arguments. However, they do need to be able to discuss and live with their differences. A couple can move beyond core arguments by learning to celebrate their differences. We will discuss this further in the third section of this book, *Solutions*.

Extramarital Affairs

Some researchers estimate that extramarital affairs occur in about half of all marriages. Given this, it is quite possible that some couples will need to deal with an extramarital affair at the same time that they are confronting cancer. Many people think that having an extramarital affair inevitably marks the end of a relationship. Others believe that the decision to have an affair is not always the product of a doomed marriage. Affairs can occur in many ways and for many reasons, and the extent to which they harm a marriage can depend on the circumstances. In fact, in some cases, an extramarital affair acts as a catalyst for a couple to closely examine their relationship and to take the necessary steps to improve it, although the healing process may take years.

Why Do People Have Affairs?

There are many reasons why a person might have an extramarital affair. Short-term affairs or "one-night stands" may simply be the result of a bad judgment call. More often though, people who turn to extramarital affairs are looking for something they have lost or never had in their marriage. In many cases, they are seeking support, love, passion, connection, or intimacy with another person.

The person engaging in an affair may view it as a way of getting some relief from tensions in the relationship. These tensions may arise from many different areas, such as chronic anger, boredom, loss, sexual problems, illness, or a family member in legal trouble. In seeking to escape such tensions, the person may have no intention of ending the marriage or committed relationship. In fact, he or she may view the affair as simply providing something that adds to what they get out of the marriage.

Sometimes affairs occur because couples have not successfully dealt with their differences in personality, temperament, and lifestyle preferences. When such differences are not addressed, it may lead to frustration and a decreased sense of connectedness. This may cause couples to develop other intimate relationships to meet their needs.

Fear of intimacy may also play a role in an extramarital affair. People who desire to maintain a comfortable level of emotional distance may seek another person to diffuse the intensity of their relationship with their spouse. If the desire for distance is strong enough, they may even hope that the affair will provoke the end of their marriage. This situation is most likely to happen after a major life change, such as when the couple is suddenly left alone after all their children have left home. Suddenly the couple must relate to each other without being distracted by the task of parenting, and this may seem impossible after years of distance.

The Effects of an Affair

Whatever the cause, an extramarital affair usually has a serious impact on a committed relationship. Many factors can affect the extent of this impact, such as:

- The length of the affair
- The frequency of the meetings
- The level of emotional connection in the affair
- The level of commitment and emotional connection in the marriage
- The level of secrecy that surrounded the affair
- The amount of sexual activity
- The prior relationship of the involved partner and the outside person
- The degree of continued contact with the outside person
- The number of past affairs
- Whether just one or both partners have had affairs
- Whether the affair was accidentally discovered or disclosed
- The history of experiences with affairs in the partners' families
- The circumstances or crises during the time of the affair
- The presence of children within the marriage

Generally speaking, affairs have more serious effects on relationships the longer they last, the greater the emotional connection is, and the more closely involved the outside person is in the couple's life (such as if it is a close friend of both partners).

Usually the discovery of an affair causes a crisis in the couple's life. The uninvolved partner may feel shock, a sense of betrayal, damaged trust and security in the relationship, anger, anxiety, and depression. Often it is difficult for this person to stop thinking about and imagining details of the affair. Even if the affair has not been discovered, the person involved in the affair may feel both happy and intensely sad at the same time. Although he or she may enjoy many aspects of the affair, this often comes along with feelings of anxiety, shame, and guilt. The involved partner feels that he or she can no longer be considered trustworthy, and that the security of the committed relationship is now precarious.

Sometimes the "secret life" element of the affair and the deceit that comes with it is more destructive than the actual sexual component. As one well-known couples therapist, Frank Pittman, M.D., expresses it, "It isn't in who you lie with, it's who you lie to" that is the root of the destruction that occurs as a result of an extramarital affair. The cumulative effects of the secrets over time can seriously increase distance between partners and separateness from each other. This blow to the intimacy in the relationship can be very difficult to recover from, and it is often particularly difficult to recover sexual intimacy following an affair.

An extramarital affair may do so much damage to a relationship that it can lead to separation and eventual divorce. One problem that often complicates the crisis caused by the affair is that the person who had the affair may become labeled as the "bad guy" in the relationship, while the person who has been betrayed is labeled as the "good guy." This is counterproductive because it places responsibility for causing and fixing the problems in the relationship solely on the bad guy's shoulders, when in fact both partners will need to work actively to heal the relationship. In Chapter 11, we explore ways couples can deal with the problems of infidelity.

Divorce

Divorce is a common reality today. It is estimated that in the United States nearly 50 percent of all marriages will end in divorce. This drastic step occurs when it seems impossible to resolve disagreements or when there seems to be no way for partners to connect in a happy or healthy way anymore. People often resort to divorce because they are simply exhausted after unsuccessfully struggling over a long period to make the relationship work. The decision of whether to end a marriage is a difficult one, however. Help is available in the form of couples counseling, which can often help couples to decide if their marriage can be saved (see Chapter 11). If a couple ultimately decides to end the marriage, counseling can also help them to separate successfully, and to work together to resolve any remaining issues.

Although at times it may seem like the only option remaining, leaving a troubled marriage does not necessarily lead to a happier life. Recent research indicates that only one out of ten people are happier after a divorce than they were before. Problems of financial loss, loneliness, and depression are common. The adjustment seems to be particularly difficult for men, who are almost twice as likely as women to commit suicide after a divorce or separation.

Cancer and Troubled Relationships

Cancer will add more strain to a relationship that is already struggling. In some cases, the cancer diagnosis may be the "straw that broke the camel's back," adding one more crisis to a list of tensions and difficulties in the marriage. Sometimes a cancer diagnosis leads a couple to consider divorce. In other cases, a person may choose to abandon the relationship because the idea that the partner may leave by dying is too difficult to bear. Other people may feel overwhelmed by the new roles of caregiving and homemaking that fall on their shoulders, particularly if these are roles in which they do not feel comfortable. Regardless of the reasons why people might consider leaving their marriage following a cancer diagnosis, it is often wise to postpone making such decisions until after the cancer crisis is past.

Emotional support is very important following a traumatic event such as a cancer diagnosis. Thus, abandonment at such a sensitive time can be especially difficult. The abandoned partner is placed in a situation in which they have to adjust to the cancer and the loss of their spouse while attempting to build a new support system. The person may eventually be able to look back and say, "It was for the best" or "We weren't going to make it anyway." Nonetheless, it can immensely add to the difficulties of coping with cancer if a person also feels alone and unsupported.

Cancer and Divorced Couples

Dealing with cancer can pose special challenges for divorced partners and their family members. Issues such as childcare, communication, and regret over lost time in the relationship may surface. If the divorce is a supportive and nonhostile one, all of the family members can often join together to meet the challenges of dealing with an ill parent or ex-partner. For example, the ex-spouse of a parent with cancer can play a very important role by taking on more of the responsibilities for caring for their children than they had before the illness.

Unfortunately, some divorced couples have very tense relationships, particularly in a new divorce or one that involves an ongoing custody dispute. In this case, dealing with cancer is just another thorny problem to resolve and work through. When tensions in the family are high, it often helps to have a third party, like a social worker or psychiatric nurse specialist, assist the family in working through the issues that arise during the illness. The outside person's perspective is helpful because it can diffuse some of the anger that is directed between the ex-partners and help them to make good, objective decisions. Often these decisions require the ex-partners to rise above their anger and resentment to provide necessary support during a time of need.

Domestic Violence

Domestic violence is a serious, and sometimes fatal, problem. In the United States, four women are beaten by their boyfriends, husbands, or ex-husbands every minute. And, although it is a less common occurrence, men can also be victims of verbal or physical abuse. Domestic violence or battering is a pattern of destructive thoughts, feelings, and actions used to establish power and control over another person through fear and intimidation. Acts of domestic violence fall into three categories:

- **Psychological battering** is an attempt to gain power and control over a person using methods other than physical force. Examples of psychological battering include verbal abuse, harassment, excessive jealousy or possessiveness, restriction of access to money, destruction of possessions, and forced isolation from friends and family.

- **Physical battering** is the use of physical force or aggression that has effects ranging from bruising to death.

- **Sexual abuse** is the use of violence or threats of violence to force someone to participate in unwanted sexual activity.

Physical Abuse

In a physically abusive relationship, the abuser, or batterer, establishes power and control over the other person through fear, intimidation, and the threat or use of violence. Batterers generally believe that they are entitled to control their partners, and they find that abuse is an effective way to maintain this control. If there are not any negative consequences for this behavior, the pattern of abuse can continue for years. Although some men are physically abused by their wives, about 95 percent of physical abuse is committed by men on their female partners. In our examples, we will assume that the batterer is a man and the victim a woman, although it should be understood that this is not always the case.

Physical abuse rarely arises out of nowhere. Usually someone who abuses his partner gives off a number of warning signs that indicate his potential to commit domestic violence. Someone who has the following characteristics may be more likely to become abusive if he:

- Feels powerless and has low self-esteem
- Suffered physical or psychological abuse as a child
- Has a father who battered the mother
- Displays violence towards other people
- Uses guns for protection from other people
- Loses his temper frequently, with little provocation
- Smashes or hits objects when angry
- Uses alcohol or drugs to excess
- Displays an unusual amount of jealousy
- Expects his partner to be present or available at all times
- Becomes enraged when he gives advice and it is not taken
- Appears to have two personalities, one kind and the other cruel
- Exhibits more cruelty or kindness than would normally be expected in a certain situation
- Becomes so angry that people avoid doing anything to upset him
- Has rigid or traditional ideas about how people should behave
- Sees women as property or objects, not as people

Batterers can have a number of other characteristics as well. They often avoid developing truly intimate relationships not only because they want to maintain complete control, but also because they may fear the emotional intensity of a close relationship. Batterers also may have other psychological issues that can contribute to their behavior, such as depression, anxiety, paranoia, impulsivity, antisocial personalities, and hostility towards the opposite sex.

Verbal Abuse

Verbal abuse can be as destructive to a relationship as physical abuse, and it can take many forms. It can involve an obvious attack or it can be more subtle and calculating. Some examples of verbal abuse include:

❥ Devaluing a partner's ideas

❥ Putting down a partner by making jokes about him or her

❥ Accusing or blaming a partner frequently

❥ Criticizing a partner frequently

❥ Calling a partner names

❥ Threatening a partner

Whatever forms the verbal abuse takes, it is often harmful to the victim's self-esteem. It also tends to result in a shutdown in communication and problem solving within the relationship.

Denying Responsibility

People who commit domestic violence are often not willing to accept responsibility for their actions. They may even try to blame their partner for the abuse. Some common methods that abusers may use to avoid taking responsibility for their actions include the following:

- **Justification:** The situation or the behavior of others is presented as an explanation for why the abuse occurred. For example, the person may say, "I threw the vase because you made me so angry."

- **Rationalization:** The abuser denies that his behavior is harmful. The person might say, "So what if I got mad and called you a couple of names? You know I didn't mean it."

- **Debilitation:** The abuser indicates that he is unable to control himself in certain situations. The person might state, "I had no other choice but to yell at you," or "I go crazy when you nag me—I can't help it."

- **Vilification:** The abuser attempts to shift blame by acting as if his partner is the villain. The person may say things such as, "I know you talked about your salary in front of my boss just to make me look bad," or "I know you tell those stories about my childhood to make me look like an idiot."

Many abusers realize deep down that their actions are wrong, but these methods of denying responsibility may help them maintain their self-image as a basically nice person. However, unless abusers are able to accept full responsibility for their actions, there is little chance that attempts to change the abusive patterns will be successful.

The Cycle of Violence

It has often been observed that domestic violence tends to occur in a pattern known as the *cycle of violence*. This pattern, which was first described by Lenore Walker, Ed.D., revolves around power and control.

In the first phase of the cycle, tension builds in the relationship, and the partner begins to sense the abuser's edginess and irritability. She tries to smooth over the rough spots and calm her partner. She denies to herself that the anger is beginning to build, and she believes that she can control the situation. During this phase, the batterer realizes that his behavior has been wrong in the past and is afraid his partner will leave him. Meanwhile, the partner is withdrawing from the abuser because she is fearful that he will explode. This withdrawal reinforces his fears of abandonment, and the tension in the relationship increases and leads to the next stage.

In the second stage, the abuser continues to get angrier until he eventually "explodes" into violence. This stage is relatively short, usually lasting a few hours to two days. Initially, the abuser may believe that he just wants to "teach a lesson" to his partner instead of hurting her. If his partner is seriously harmed by the abuse, he may then attempt to avoid responsibility for his actions by focusing on how he was provoked into them. The woman may or may not fight back in defense. The victim is often embarrassed or ashamed by the abuse. This may lead her to deny the extent of her injuries and to keep the evidence of the abuse hidden from friends and family.

Both partners welcome the next stage of forgiveness and reconciliation. During this stage, the abuser is remorseful and fears that his partner might abandon him. He may promise not to abuse his partner ever again and truly believes what he is saying. This sincerity may add a sense of credibility to his promise. Furthermore, his partner may have her own reasons for wanting to believe him. She may remember the honeymoon phase of their relationship and hope that they can recapture these good times. Often the abuser reinforces this fantasy by bringing home flowers and candy, helping with housework, and generally "turning over a new leaf." The abuser may also appeal to her caregiving instincts by telling her that he cannot live without her. With the bad times put behind them, they both look forward to a happy future until the tension begins to rebuild, and the cycle is repeated.

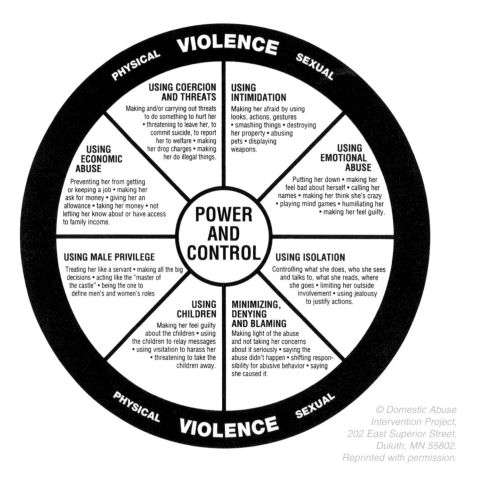

Is Your Partner Abusive or Potentially Abusive?

The following is a checklist for assessing if your partner is abusive or potentially abusive.

➤ Does your partner:
- Embarrass you or make fun of you in front of your friends or family?
- Belittle your accomplishments or goals?
- Make you feel like you are unable to make decisions?
- Use intimidation or threats to gain compliance?
- Tell you that you are nothing without him?
- Treat you roughly—grab, push, pinch, shove, or hit you?
- Call you several times a night or show up to make sure you are where you said you would be?
- Use drugs or alcohol as an excuse for saying hurtful things or abusing you?
- Blame you for how he feels or acts?
- Pressure you sexually for things you aren't ready for?
- Make you feel that there is no way out of the relationship?
- Prevent you from doing things you want—like spending time with your friends or family?
- Try to keep you from leaving after a fight or leave you somewhere after a fight to "teach you a lesson"?

➤ Do you:
- Sometimes feel scared of how your partner will act?
- Constantly make excuses to other people for your partner's behavior?
- Believe that you can help your partner change if only you changed something about yourself?
- Try not to do anything that would cause conflict or make your partner angry?
- Feel like no matter what you do, your partner is never happy with you?
- Always do what your partner wants you to do instead of what you want?
- Stay with your partner because you are afraid of what your partner would do if you broke up?

Reprinted with permission of the National Coalition Against Domestic Violence. Adapted from Reaching and Teaching Teens to Stop Violence. Nebraska Domestic Violence and Sexual Assault Coalition, Lincoln, NE.

If you responded yes to any of these questions, it is important for you to discuss your situation with somebody you trust, such as your doctor. Abuse usually continues until people take action to stop it. In Chapter 11, we discuss some specific ways to confront domestic violence.

The Abuse Victim

Many people who have not themselves lived with abuse wonder why anybody would choose to stay with an abusive partner. There are many reasons why an otherwise rational person would make what seems to be such an obviously destructive choice. The victim may choose to stay because she:

- Has low self-esteem and believes that she deserves this treatment or couldn't attract a partner that would not abuse her
- Believes, based on her own experiences growing up, that abuse is a normal part of a relationship
- Believes that she cannot leave because she is financially dependent on her partner
- Does not want to face the financial and other difficulties of being a single parent
- Fears that the abuser will find her and hurt her
- Loves or feels committed to her partner
- Is too embarrassed to admit that she's being abused
- Believes that the abuser is basically a good man who wants to change
- Believes that the abuse is the result of alcohol or drug use, and doesn't reflect the abuser's true personality
- Believes that she can control the situation
- Doesn't feel there is a safe place to go, often as a result of gradual isolation from family and friends

To the person involved in an abusive relationship, any of the above may seem to be good enough reasons to stay. However, domestic violence is not only damaging to a relationship—it can also be very dangerous to the victim. Physical abuse tends to get worse over time, increasing in both frequency and severity. When the victim finally decides to leave the abusive relationship, this can enrage the abusive partner, making the situation particularly dangerous.

PAULA HAS RECENTLY BEEN DIAGNOSED WITH BREAST CANCER and is undergoing radiation therapy treatments. When the team examines her in preparation her for her simulation (when they draw the radiation markings on the body), they notice bruises on her back. Paula denies her husband is hitting her. Instead, she states she ran into the door at home. After the team has been treating her for a few weeks, she misses two appointments without calling. When she returns to the clinic, she has fresh bruises on her back, chest, and arms. The social worker at the clinic talks with Paula, and she admits that her husband has been hitting her for years. The social worker calls Adult Protective Services and refers Paula to the local domestic violence organization. They help Paula find temporary housing and ensure that she has consistent transportation for her daily radiation treatments. The social worker will continue to work with Paula until her problems are resolved.

Alcoholism or Drug Problems

Alcohol is the drug of choice in the United States. It contributes to many of our society's problems, including automobile accidents, child abuse, rape, suicide, and other forms of violence. It also contributes to many physical problems, including cancer. Alcoholism is a major risk factor in the development of head and neck cancers (cancers of the mouth, pharynx, larynx, and esophagus). Alcohol also increases the risk of developing breast cancer. Compared with nondrinkers, women who consume one alcoholic drink a day have a slight increase in risk, and those who have two to five drinks daily have about one and a half times the risk of women who drink no alcohol.

In addition to contributing to these other problems, alcoholism can wreak havoc with intimate relationships. Alcoholics often lose their spouse, children, other family members, and friends as a result of their drinking.

What Is Alcoholism?

Alcoholism is a chronic disease that is influenced by both genetic and environmental factors. Alcoholism tends to get more severe over time, and it is often eventually fatal. Most alcoholics either sometimes or always: 1) have difficulty controlling their drinking; 2) think about alcohol a lot; 3) use alcohol

Do You Have a Problem with Alcohol?

The following list of questions, developed by Alcoholics Anonymous, may help you evaluate whether you or a family member may be an alcoholic. If you (or your family member) answer yes to four or more of these questions, then you (or your family member) may have a drinking problem:

1. Have you ever decided to stop drinking for a week or so, but only lasted for a couple of days?

2. Do you wish people would mind their own business about your drinking and stop telling you what to do?

3. Have you ever switched from one kind of drink to another in the hope that this would keep you from getting drunk?

4. Have you had to have an eye-opener upon awakening during the past year? Do you need a drink to get the day started, or to stop shaking?

5. Do you envy people who can drink without getting into trouble?

6. Have you had problems connected with drinking during the past year?

7. Has your drinking caused trouble at home?

8. Do you ever try to get "extra" drinks at a party because you do not get enough?

9. Do you tell yourself you can stop drinking any time you want to, even though you keep getting drunk when you don't mean to?

10. Have you missed days of work or school because of drinking?

11. Do you have "blackouts"?

12. Have you ever felt that your life would be better if you did not drink?

even though it causes them problems; and 4) are distorted in their thinking, and in particular, are in denial about their drinking problem. Often this denial of the extent of the alcohol problem is also shared by family members of the alcoholic.

Alcoholism and Relationships

Alcoholism can affect relationships in many ways, both directly and indirectly. Alcoholism can contribute to several other problems that can seriously harm family relationships, including extramarital affairs, depression, domestic violence, incest, sexual problems, work problems, and compulsive behaviors such as gambling or overeating.

In addition to these indirect effects, alcoholism can also directly affect how family members relate to each other. When one partner is having difficulty with alcohol, the other partner often does his or her best to prevent the drinking from causing problems for the family. Alcohol becomes a factor that needs to be considered in almost every aspect of daily life. For example, a family may completely change their holiday rituals as a result of the alcoholic's drinking patterns. If it appears that the alcoholic will be drinking, the family may decide to hold their dinner earlier, put the children to bed earlier, and ensure that the drinker does not drive.

Over time, the alcoholic becomes less and less responsible for his or her actions, while the partner handles more and more of the family responsibilities. Often these responsibilities include taking steps to limit the damage caused by the drinking, such as making excuses when the alcoholic misses work. Although such actions may limit the short-term problems caused by the drinking, in the long run they also enable the drinking to continue.

As the partner gradually becomes the caretaker of the couple, the alcoholic may begin to feel worthless and useless. Meanwhile, the partner can begin to feel overburdened and resentful. Due to this stressful situation, the partner of the alcoholic may experience physical and psychological problems. Unfortunately, because alcoholism usually progresses over many years, the habits that are formed in these years are hard to break, even if they are recognized as being unhealthy. Often this destructive pattern of caretaking continues for years.

When both partners are alcoholic, their relationship and their lives may stay in "ordered chaos"; that is, although drinking causes some problems for both of them, they function well enough to maintain their lifestyle. In this situation, children often assume the role of caretaker to both parents. As a result, the children not only grow up without effective parenting, but they also lose a part of their childhood because of the adult roles they are forced to play. In Chapter 11, we explore treatment options and help for both the person with a dependence on alcohol or other drugs and his or her partner.

SINCE JACK WAS DIAGNOSED WITH ESOPHAGEAL CANCER, he has decided to seek help for his alcoholism by entering a substance abuse program. He decides to join Alcoholics Anonymous. For the duration of his chemotherapy, Jack does not feel like drinking and has attended as many A.A. meetings as he physically can. He knows that his cancer diagnosis was a wakeup call, and he intends to heed it. His wife, Janet, however, is skeptical. She has been living with his drinking for the past twenty-five years. She regularly called his boss about his coming in late, or being sick and not coming in at all. She has put him to bed drunk more times than she cares to count. She has seen Jack try to quit before, and she doesn't believe that this time is going to be any different. Janet doesn't believe that Jack will stop until he literally drinks himself to death. She will believe it when she sees it.

Although we have focused on alcohol here, the abuse of any other drug has similar effects on relationships. Illicit drug abuse may also cause additional problems, such as legal and financial troubles. As with alcoholism, substance use replaces normal, healthy coping mechanisms and becomes the focus for the addicted. Regardless of the drug of choice, the destruction of lives and relationships is often the result.

As we have seen in this chapter, relationships can be affected by a variety of problems. Although these problems are completely separate from the experience of having cancer, they often can add a great deal of stress to a cancer patient's life. The good news, though, is that there are ways to solve many of these problems, or at least to cope with them in a healthy manner. We will provide advice on dealing with these problems in Section 3 of this book, *Solutions*.

Chapter Seven

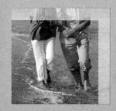

Lifestyle
Factors

In this chapter, we discuss the background for your relationship—your family composition and lifestyle—that may influence your experiences as a couple dealing with cancer. Specifically, we will discuss parenting, blended families, dual-career couples, and same-sex couples. Each of these lifestyles can affect how you cope with cancer, in ways that are positive or negative. This chapter will help you understand how each of these factors is likely to challenge you and your partner. In Chapter 11, we will discuss more specific strategies and resources to help you cope with the challenges we identify here.

Parenting

After having children, couples must renegotiate their relationship in many ways. The boundaries of the family unit must expand to include the children, each of them with unique personalities and challenges. Balancing the couple identity with the parental role is not always easy. Sometimes couples begin to lose their "coupleness" in the process of parenting, and the children become the primary focus of their lives. However, your closeness with your partner must remain intact for the relationship to flourish while raising children. We briefly visited these issues in Chapter 4 and return to explore them in more detail here.

One of the challenges parenting introduces for couples is style differences. The style differences between the two of you also may become particularly apparent as you raise your children together. Your style of parenting may have been learned during your own childhood. Naturally when you and your partner are trying to serve as a "united front" in guiding and disciplining the children, the differences in your respective experiences can become all too obvious.

Children also bring deeper meaning to the lives of couples. For many couples, having children and being parents is the most enjoyable part of their relationship. Although children require a lot of attention and work, they also provide joy, stability, and purpose. While parenting children and talking about the mutual endeavor, partners may bond in their shared joys and worries. Having children is immensely challenging, and as such, represents a growth experience for many people. Each parent may see the other now not only as a significant other, but also as a teammate in parenting. In a successful relationship, couples are able to make these adjustments and allow a child to come into the family.

For many couples, especially during the cancer experience, children are an anchor that motivates both parents, spurring them to get up in the morning and cope with life's realities. Having children and being obligated to be parents, no matter what is going on personally, can help to keep a couple grounded and engaged in life.

In traditional, nonadoptive families, the birth experience and early parenting are often especially life-altering for the new mother, who physically experienced giving birth to the child and (if she nurses) serves as the primary physical caregiver in the early months. The mother's experience may be somewhat different in couples who adopt a child or do not breast-feed.

In couples in which the mother is the primary caregiver, the father may feel somewhat deserted by the mother's focus on the demanding new baby. There is some evidence that in couples with traditional parenting roles, the father's adjustment to parenthood may be particularly important for the couple's overall adjustment. In such situations, helping the father and baby form a bond, and ensuring that the couple maintains a close enough connection, is important and can be difficult at times.

Parenting and Cancer

In Chapter 2, we briefly mentioned the challenge of communicating with children about cancer. We now resume our discussion of this issue in more detail. Parents must cope with both their own and their children's emotional reactions to cancer. Cancer disrupts family routines that normally ground most children. Parents who lived separately after a divorce may reunite to help cope with the cancer. One or both parents may not be working, and there may be financial concerns. Children may have a variety of substitute caregivers. All of these changes may confuse and upset children, and therefore pose a challenge to parents who are trying to help them cope.

Develop a Game Plan for Talking with Your Children

Before you talk with your children about the cancer diagnosis, it is a good idea to sit down with your partner and come up with a plan about how to share this information with your children. Usually you have some time to do this before it becomes essential to talk with your children. That gives you and your partner time and space to talk, cry, and worry together about the news. You can also put childcare plans into place and further explore any household changes that the children will need to be told.

Plan to speak with your children during a time that will be quiet and without interruptions, and be prepared for what you will say. Your game plan for talking to your children should include a "who," "what," "when," and "how."

Who. Both parents should sit down with the children to talk about the cancer. The decision as to who will say what will vary according to your personalities and parental roles and your children's needs. If Mom is the usual spokesperson, she may be the best person to speak first. The most important thing is that both partners participate in the discussion. That will reassure the children that you can both discuss the cancer and that either of you is open to further discussion.

What. You and your partner should prepare ahead of time what each of you will say to the children. What you tell them should be the truth about the diagnosis and treatment, simplified to a degree that is appropriate to their ages. Talk with your partner about exactly what words you would like to use.

Discuss the treatment and how it will impact their lives. You may have a pre-arranged plan that you will need to help them prepare for emotionally, such as your plans for their care when a parent is hospitalized or otherwise unavailable.

When. Both partners need to agree on an acceptable time after diagnosis to tell the rest of the family, including the children. While there is some flexibility in this decision, it should be done before other family members and friends start talking about it. You would hate for your children to hear the news by mistake before you have had a chance to sit down and tell them.

How. As a couple, you should agree on the tone to set when talking with the children. You can give simple explanations and reassure them that you are still in charge. Children need to feel safe and know that their world will basically remain intact.

Keep Communication Flowing

Children tend to accept what they are told at face value, and they generally believe what you tell them. So, they need to be told the truth about what is happening in a straightforward manner at a level they can understand. Protecting children from the truth can actually do more harm than good. If you try to keep big news a secret, children can sense something is happening anyway. They will either notice a change in your mood or overhear you or others talking. It is much more worrisome to children to know something is wrong without crucial information than to have all of the facts up front. Children often imagine the worst.

> PETER, WHO WAS A CAREGIVER FOR HIS WIFE, said, "Telling your children is the hardest part. It is essential that you think through what you are going to say, as the words and emotions will have a significant impact on how the children will react. The calmer you are, the less frightened they will be...[Still,] as calm as we were, the revelation of cancer was a huge shock to our kids and was met with fear and tears. It is essential that kids are reassured that their parents are going to do everything possible in the way of treatment, that they are still deeply loved and always will be, and if necessary, assured that none of this is their fault."

How to Explain Cancer to Younger Children

One way to think about cancer and what it means is to compare it to a garden. Gardens grow herbs, flowers, and vegetables. But weeds also grow in a garden and may keep the good plants from growing. Cancer cells in a person's body are like the weeds in the garden. They can harm the good cells and keep them from growing. When weeds come up in a garden, they are pulled out, dug up, and removed in some way. Cancer cells must also be removed from the body. Sometimes surgery is used to take the cancer cells out, too. There are other ways to kill the cancer cells. These ways are called chemotherapy or radiation therapy. These treatments help rid the body of the cancer cells, just like chopping out the weeds helps get them out of the garden.

Younger children sometimes believe the world revolves around them. They may mistakenly think that they are in some way responsible for bad things that happen, including a parent's illness. The guilt that comes from this mistaken belief can be quite a burden, so it is better to be honest about the facts of the situation.

Much like adults, children's reactions typically include shock, disbelief, and denial. Fear and anxiety are common, along with sadness, anger, and guilt. Children—especially younger ones—sometimes express their anxiety with physical symptoms or other behavior changes, such as sleep problems, eating problems, or reverting to more childish behavior.

You are the best source of information for your children. Your children should be given information from you—not their teachers, neighbors, or peers. Be as honest and sensitive as you can. Answer whatever questions children have as openly and clearly as possible, and allow them to react emotionally to what's happening. In this way you will reinforce one of many life lessons on how to cope with stress.

As with the other people in your life, communicating with children about cancer is not a one-time event. It is a process that continues throughout the illness. Children may be overwhelmed by the effort to absorb all of the information at once, and—just like you—they may need information repeated or explained differently. Keep children posted throughout the treatment and the time after treatment.

Trish is a thirty-six-year-old mother of two children, Chad and Sara, ages six and eight. She was diagnosed with stage III breast cancer six months ago. Prior to her diagnosis, she worked as a part-time freelance writer for several local publications. Her husband, Steve, works for a major downtown accounting firm, so Trish has stayed at home to care for the children after school.

WHEN TRISH WAS FIRST DIAGNOSED (after discovering a breast lump), she and Steve were totally shocked. They spent a full three weeks deciding on treatment options and doctors, and then planned how to tell the kids.

The discussion was short and to the point. Trish explained that she had breast cancer, pointing to her breast in the correct location. She compared the cancer to a "sick spot" like a scrape on the knee, except it was inside the body. She would be getting medicine that might make her feel sick and tired. Steve then talked about how he would be helping out while Mommy was not feeling well. They both talked about how the children would get to their soccer games, and that the whole family would go to church on the weekend as usual. Trish told Chad and Sara that they had nothing to do with causing her illness, and that it wasn't anyone's fault that she had cancer. They both expressed their hope that all would be well once the treatment was completed and the cancer was gone.

The children expressed their reactions appropriately in their usual ways. Chad gave his mommy a hug and ran off to draw her a picture. Sara cuddled with her mother for a while, then called a friend to come over.

At first, as Trish went through surgery and started chemotherapy, her husband took some time off to help her manage her recovery and the home responsibilities. As the weeks went on, he needed to return to work and she asked friends to help with the kids, transportation, and food. There were times when she needed to act a little more energetic than she felt around the kids. It hurt when they said, "Mommy, you're always tired." It was a hard time, but the kids never seemed to be too terribly upset by it all. They asked questions about her hair loss, but seemed to take most things in stride. Trish and Steve tried to make sure that one of them was always available to the children.

Questions That Are Difficult to Answer

Parents often avoid conversations about cancer with their children because they're afraid of answering difficult questions. Thinking in advance about questions that may be asked, and how to respond to them, will help in being prepared. The answers to all questions should be honest, but as optimistic as the situation allows. For example, "This is a serious illness, but I am getting the best possible treatment, and the doctor thinks I am responding very well." When optimism is not realistic, parents need to acknowledge how difficult it is to live with uncertainty and to emphasize their determination to confront whatever happens together as a family.

"Are you going to die?" This is the question that all parents dread. The question about the possibility of death is the one that causes the most distress to everyone in families coping with cancer. Some children may not ask about it up front, but this worry is undoubtedly on their mind as it is on everyone else's. By around age eight, children can begin to understand death as a permanent state. It is a good idea to rehearse how you are going to respond to this. There are some things you should realize before you answer this question. First, this is a scary question for children to ask, and they may never ask it directly. Children will need more assistance than adults to deal with this issue because they have less life experience and rely upon adults to learn how to cope with painful events. Although it is painful to talk about, it is much better than being silent in the long run.

You will need to set the stage that you and the family will be living with cancer. Focusing the family on how to live with cancer, not how to die with it, is a constructive approach.

What You Can Say

Here are some examples of what other parents have said in response to the question about death:

❧ Sometimes people do die from cancer. I'm not expecting that to happen because the doctors have told me they have very good treatments these days.

❧ Many people are cured of cancer these days—that's why I'm getting treatment.

❧ The doctors have told me that my chances of being cured are very good. I think we should believe them until they tell us otherwise. I'll let you know if that changes.

❧ There is no way to know right now what's going to happen until I get some treatment. I think we should feel positive about things for now, and hopefully we will feel even better in the future.

❧ Years ago, people often died from cancer because treatments weren't as good. Now there are a lot more choices of treatment, and the outlook for many cancers is much more hopeful.

❧ They don't know a lot about the kind of cancer I have, but I'm certainly going to give it my best.

❧ My cancer is a tough illness to treat, but I'm going to work hard at getting better. We just don't know what is going to happen. The most important thing is that we stick together as a family and let each other know what each of us is thinking. If you can't stop worrying, I want you to tell me because there are things we can do to feel better.

❧ I don't think I'm going to die. None of us knows for sure. But I'm going to do everything the doctors ask me to do so that doesn't happen.

Here are some examples of other important questions children may ask:

- Can I or someone else catch it?
- Is it inherited?
- Did I cause it?
- Is it going to hurt?
- Is cancer a punishment?

- Does radiation make people radioactive?
- What is going to happen to me?

Being prepared to answer such questions ahead of time can help when you are talking with your children. While these questions may not be asked directly, these are things children think about when a parent gets cancer. Although you will not know the answers to all of these questions, especially when you are first diagnosed, these issues need to be discussed at some point in your experience.

Helping Children Cope

A cancer diagnosis may be the first crisis you have faced as a couple. The way you cope as parents with the emotional and lifestyle disruptions of cancer will set the stage for how your children will deal with them. Children often react more to how parents behave than to what they actually say.

Unfortunately, parents probably cannot offer the kind of reassurance they would like to at the beginning of their experience with cancer. This is because no one really knows at that point how the patient will respond to treatment. In spite of this, there are things that parents can do to help their children begin coping with this new reality. Parents can say that even though they can't see into the future, they can promise that the children will be taken care of. If the parent is feeling sick, they will arrange for someone else to fill in. The most important psychological issue for children is their own sense of security and safety. Children often need frequent reassurance that they'll still be loved and safe, no matter what happens.

Cancer and its treatment require many absences from home, and young-sters are often left in the care of others for periods of time. One of the things children get mad about is feeling left out or neglected. Some feel that they don't get as much attention as before, and this may actually be the case at times. It can help if you listen to them and acknowledge these feelings. Parents have a lot on their minds at this time, which may not leave much time for children—especially if parents are making frequent trips to the clinic or hospital. Children need reassurance that they are not being abandoned, and that their parents are always going to make sure they are okay, no matter what happens.

Call in the Troops!

Now is the time to overcome your own reluctance to ask for help. No one can manage the cancer experience alone. You and your family shouldn't have to either. When a friend or acquaintance states, "If there is anything I can do...," have your list ready. Most people are eager to help someone in this situation and will appreciate your specific suggestions. If it's difficult to do it for yourself, think of how your children may benefit if you show them how to ask for and receive help appropriately. When helping the children cope with cancer, you and your partner may need to turn to each other for help too. Sometimes your partner may have just the right touch with the children at moments when you feel spent, and vice versa. Grandparents or other adults with whom the children feel close may also be helpful in this regard.

Here are some specific suggestions for how you might help your children deal with the cancer in the family:

- **Talk to your children's teachers.** If a parent informs the teacher of the family's situation, teachers can be prepared for problems that may occur in school as a result. Even if the outlook for the person with cancer is good, tell teachers about the situation. They can be an extra source of support for your children. They can also provide information about how your children are coping.

- **Develop a support network for your children.** Seeing to your children's emotional and physical needs can be extraordinarily difficult in the face of illness-related absences or disability, especially if the other parent has to work extra hours to compensate for lost earnings or increased costs. You may need to call on friends and relatives to provide childcare.

- **Maintain your children's normal routines.** Allow children to take part in their usual activities in and out of school as much as possible. Routines give children the security they need to continue their social and intellectual development. Adolescents in particular need to continue to spend time with their peers and have their privacy so that they can explore the world in preparation for adulthood.

- **Continue your usual discipline with your children.** Children need to know their limits, especially at times of disruption. Discipline problems can arise during a stressful time, either because children may attempt to use unwanted behaviors get the attention they feel is missing, or because they don't yet know how to express their emotional reactions to stress. The ideal way to respond is to combine your usual method of limit-setting for inappropriate behavior with reasonable acknowledgment of any painful feelings of anger, sadness, or anxiety that may have contributed to your child's undesired behavior. You can acknowledge your child's feelings without tolerating inappropriate behavior.

- **Involve your children in projects to help.** Give children something to do if they want to be involved, whether it's caring for household pets, helping with meals, or keeping track of schedules. Giving them practical tasks can help them feel useful and more in control of the situation.

- **Ask your children what they think.** When dealing with an illness in the family, asking for your children's input in resolving the logistical and emotional issues that emerge in the household may provide a much-needed sense of competence.

- **Allow your children to have fun without feeling guilty.** Encourage children to keep doing the things they did before you or your partner were diagnosed, such as going out with friends, playing games, and joining extracurricular activities. These are the same sorts of activities that help adults cope with difficult times.

Blended Families

About half of all married people have had a previous marriage. A blended family is defined as one in which children live some, most, or all of the time with two married adults, one of whom is not a biological parent. This is the fastest growing type of family composition in the United States. By the year 2010, it is expected that in the United States there will be more blended families (also called stepfamilies) than any other kind of family.

The bond between the biological or original parent and the child is usually stronger than the new relationship between the child and stepparent. Children sometimes feel torn between loyalty to their new family and to their former family. The situation can be further complicated if you and your partner have not yet developed harmonious parental styles with each other.

Stepmothers have a unique challenge. In many households, the role of the stepmother is to have primary responsibility for childcare and household tasks. In families in which they have this role, they may interact more with stepchildren and tend to be the enforcers of rules. They must overcome centuries of "wicked stepmother" folklore. Therefore, stepmothers sometimes feel particularly sensitive about their ability to bond with children. In many families, stepfathers may go through the same feelings. Sometimes the child in a blended family simply needs a scapegoat for anger, fear, frustration, and disappointment. Stepmothers sometimes play this role, as do stepfathers. In general, stepparents may find it difficult to decide the right amount of authority to exert in the new family, especially if all of the children in the blended household are the partner's offspring.

The Special Challenges

Despite the *Brady Bunch* stereotype, this type of "instant family" can create significant stress for parents and children. Blended families all have a history of significant loss. With the breakup of the former relationship, family members' dreams for their future are permanently changed. If there is a geographical move with the separation, there may even be the loss of close friends.

When cancer enters the picture, the family is changed again. Once again, everyone in the family has to adjust to a new lifestyle and changing routines.

Since the children have already experienced loss of their original nuclear family, their previous fears and anxieties may affect their coping now.

During this time, the entire family is likely to feel anxious and unsettled, and the emotions in the household may be strained. In spite of this, parents can help by trying to keep as much of their children's lives the same as possible, since children thrive on routine and a sense of security. This may sound like a tall order when the adults are feeling anxious, but it is worth making the effort. At the same time, it is a good idea to prepare children for certain changes that will need to be made in the family routine during treatment.

The impact that cancer has on a blended family depends on how bonded or connected they are to each other. There is a process that occurs over time as a blended family becomes a unit. During the early stage, stepfamilies may have unrealistic ideas about blending together. Sometimes stepparents want to rescue their partners and children, so they immediately try to adore their stepchildren and heal the broken family.

As the couple begins to form a partnership, they try to fit their families together. This is hard because the pieces they are trying to fit together are from different molds. Both parents and children may experience feelings of jealousy, resentment, confusion, and inadequacy. Any bonds of love that form between the child and stepparent are not instantaneous, but develop over time. Until he or she has established a bond with the children, the stepparent often needs to play the role of "camp counselor" or friend, but not parental disciplinarian.

Setting up household rules that all family members can agree upon can be helpful. If there has been a consensus on household roles, it is easier for stepparents to enforce the house rules without feeling like the "bad guy." Younger children may have an easier time than older children in adjusting to changes in their environment. Recent research suggests that young adolescents, between the ages of ten and fourteen, may have the most difficult time adjusting to a stepfamily. Older adolescents may be more removed from their parents as a normal part of their growth and development, whereas younger children may find it easier to adapt to an addition to the family. In Chapter 11, we will offer more guidelines for helping blended families cope.

The Benefits

There are many advantages to the blended family. Partners who have a new opportunity to meet their own intimacy needs or get some relief from single parenting may have the most to gain. Another positive aspect of blended families is the opportunity to be exposed to a wider array of people and experiences. When the new relationship is a supportive one, the children then have an opportunity to observe a positive model for couple relationships.

There also may be more adults available to the child than before the new union was formed. Stepparents often bring objectivity to the blended family that is missing in the biological nuclear family, in which relationships may be more emotional and intense. Adults who have had a previous relationship fail are often motivated to make this relationship work, which may provide extra sticking power. Since more flexibility is required in stepparenting, there is often more cooperation and negotiation. And because flexibility is also required of stepchildren, they may learn to "go with the flow."

When one parent is diagnosed with cancer, stepfamilies often have more people available to fill in. Stepparents, grown children from this or a prior relationship, extended family, or ex-partners in some cases, may help with the household duties, preparing meals, running errands, taking trips to the hospital, and shuttling the children back and forth to their extracurricular events. This can help the family continue many of their regular activities. Cancer may actually become a focal point that helps the family rally together and develop more closeness and intimacy.

Dual-Career Couples

A dual-career couple is one in which both partners pursue jobs that are personally fulfilling, that have an established "career ladder," and which require a high degree of commitment. Decisions within the couple are based on what works for both careers. Over the past forty years since the beginning of the women's movement, women have entered the work force in greater numbers, increasing the number of dual-career couples.

Recent research suggests that the dual-career lifestyle can be stressful to couples, and to women in particular. There are several stresses that contribute to that reality. When both partners have busy careers, they each have work and home responsibilities. Simply by virtue of having two jobs there are more tasks required of both partners in these situations. There may be more focus on "getting stuff done" than the quality of the interactions in their lives.

Commonly, the female partner of a dual-career couple begins what could be called the "second shift" when she returns home from work. This work consists of housework and childcare. If both partners do not agree on how these tasks should be divided, it can cause major conflicts in the relationship.

Many dual-career couples are high achievers. They may do a great job at work and at home, but often their intimate lives suffer as a result. Sometimes, both partners compete with each other for higher status and stronger job performance. When this happens, it does not create a warm, supportive environment. Moreover, since dual-career couples often do not have a great deal of time for socializing, supportive friendships may suffer as well. Tensions and guilt resulting from having to leave children in day care may also contribute to stress for dual-career partners. All of these factors can affect how well a couple copes with the additional stress of cancer.

Such couples often have less scheduling flexibility—a problem that is compounded by the complexities of cancer treatment. This necessitates more discussion, arranging, and negotiation. Sometimes, couples complain that there is little or no time left for intimacy after this working out of schedules and duties. It is often difficult to anticipate and manage priorities when unexpected events occur, such as when a partner is diagnosed with cancer. In these situations, the little free time that remains is generally spent focusing on treatment-related concerns, leaving even less time for intimacy.

JOAN IS AN ATTORNEY FOR A LARGE HIGH-PROFILE FIRM. She was diagnosed with breast cancer just after she was promoted to partner status. She worked an average of seventy hours a week to get to this position in the company. Her husband Jim is an advertising executive on the fast track in his career, and he also puts in many overtime hours. Often, the only quality time Jim and Joan had together was on Sunday afternoons. They reserved that time to relax, go to the movies, or just be together. When Joan was going through chemotherapy, however, Jim cut back on some of his hours at work during the week to help Joan. That meant that he had to go into the office on Sunday afternoons to catch up on his regular workload. They soon lost their feeling of emotional connection as they became focused on the practical needs related to treatment.

In spite of these challenges, there are benefits to the dual-career lifestyle. Often these partners have a multitude of interests and lead stimulating and productive lives. Sharing these experiences with each other lends an air of excitement to the relationship. Couples who have two careers are also generally more financially secure. Their quality of life may be better, and there is less financial stress. Extra income helps with the many tasks of the dual-career household, including housework and childcare. One partner may also have flexibility to consider a career shift if he or she can depend on someone else for financial support during the transition (see Chapter 11 for more information on how dual-career couples cope).

Same-Sex Couples

In a generally homophobic society, there are many social pressures for gay and lesbian couples. Discrimination may occur in schools, churches, housing agencies, businesses, and employment practices. It is often difficult to decide whether to declare your lifestyle openly in the work setting. Acknowledging being gay at work may be especially risky for people who work with children, such as teaching or childcare. Many people are not comfortable risking discrimination and remain "in the closet."

For many same-sex couples, there are other troubling challenges in their lives in addition to the social stigma. Same-sex partners may not have the same legal rights as heterosexual couples. And marriage is not legally recognized for gay or lesbian couples in the United States. This may have implications when one partner has been diagnosed with cancer, since inheritance funds, paid leave for family illness or death, tax return filing, reduced insurance family plans, decision making for an incompetent partner, or shared parental rights are all affected by legal marital status. Some of these problems can be circumvented by legally appointing the other partner as power of attorney who makes the health care decisions.

Same-sex couples also face the same problems faced by heterosexual couples with regard to communication, closeness, and sexuality. However, there may be unique challenges that compound these problems. Keeping secrets, the lack of a traditional commitment ceremony and legal status, and the lack of family support are just a few. The quality and availability of a support network can make a difference in the ability of same-sex couples to cope with a diagnosis of cancer. Many have separated from their families who are uncomfortable with their lifestyle. Therefore, the support that most couples would depend on during this time of need is not available for many gay couples. Gay and lesbian couples often choose larger urban settings that offer resources and a community to help with this isolation (see Chapter 11 for ways same-sex couples can get support).

SECTION 3
Solutions

In the previous section, we mainly focused on the challenges couples face when confronting cancer. Lifestyle issues, emotions and intimacy, and problems such as divorce, infidelity, and alcohol abuse, present challenges for couples, even when both partners are in good medical health. When one partner is suddenly diagnosed with cancer on top of these problems, life can seem very overwhelming.

Can you grow through the experience of this serious illness together, or will it break your relationship? In this section, we look at some strategies and resources to help you overcome the various challenges we have been discussing. By learning new ways to cope, as well as using the strengths you already have, you can work through the turmoil and become closer through the crisis.

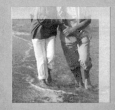

Chapter Eight

Improving
Communication

Throughout this book, we have discussed the importance of good communication for dealing with various problems and for building happy, long-lasting relationships. Unfortunately, good communication does not always come easily, and it can be complicated by many factors.

Partners have different personalities, family histories, and goals—all of which can influence communication styles. With each partner coming from a different perspective, it can be difficult to understand the other's position. When a couple is faced with an emotional and stressful situation such as cancer, communication can become even more trying. Fortunately, there are many steps that a couple can take to improve their communication. We will explore several helpful strategies in this chapter.

Communication and Cancer

Communication is essential in overcoming the challenges that arise in any relationship. With the many additional challenges that a couple faces when confronting cancer, the need for good communication becomes even stronger. Unfortunately, cancer itself can sometimes lead to communication problems. Partners often have different ways of dealing with cancer, and their coping styles affect how they relate with each other. As a result, even partners who communicated well before the cancer may suddenly find it difficult to talk about their complex and intense feelings.

Sometimes communication problems arise because each partner needs something different from a conversation. For example, the person with cancer may want to talk about the progression of the illness, but the healthy partner may not be ready to acknowledge what is happening. Or the partner without cancer may be afraid, while the ill person is more positive and hopeful. In situations like these, it helps if couples listen closely to each other and try to understand each other's perspectives.

Cancer can also disrupt the openness of the communication between partners. Partners often feel protective of each other and try to hide their upsetting thoughts or feelings. It is especially common for partners to have difficulty talking about death because they do not want to sound like they have given up hope. In more extreme cases, a person may try to avoid talking about the cancer altogether. In any of these situations, conversation can become stiff and awkward. Although it may be done with good intentions, withholding or denying genuine feelings creates distance in the relationship and allows stress and tension to build. In contrast, open and honest communication can help a couple solve the problems they face and increase the level of mutual understanding and support in their relationship.

Build Basic Communication Skills

Good communication involves not only openly sharing thoughts and feelings with your partner, but also actively listening to your partner's thoughts and feelings. Like many other aspects of a good relationship, this takes effort from both partners. It also requires skills that you may or may not have when you enter a relationship. Regardless of where you start from, however, good communication skills can be learned with practice.

Look at the World Through Your Partner's Eyes

The ability to understand your partner's point of view is central to good communication. The best way to do this is to ensure that you really listen to what your partner is saying. This takes some effort, particularly during an argument. When people argue, they can be so focused on figuring out what to say to prove themselves right that they ignore the meaning of what their partner is saying. This can result in people talking past each other instead of communicating effectively.

Following some basic "speaker" and "listener" rules is a good way to prevent a communication breakdown. When you are the speaker, you should try to create a situation in which your partner doesn't need to direct mental energy being defensive instead of listening to you. Here are some ways you can minimize defensive responses:

- Describe the problem without blaming the other person.
- Stay on the specific topic without bringing in other hot issues.
- Talk about how you feel, using sentences beginning with "I."
- Avoid criticism or insults.

The person listening should focus on understanding what the speaker is saying, even if he or she doesn't agree with it. It also helps to give the speaker non-verbal signals that what is being said is interesting and important to you. Here are some hints for improving your listening skills:

- Pay close and courteous attention.
- Make eye contact with the speaker, and avoid looking at distractions like the television.
- Try not to cross your arms as it can make you appear defensive or uninterested.
- Don't interrupt, no matter how much you want to.
- Ask questions if you do not understand what the speaker is saying.
- Before you respond, try rephrasing what your partner said, and then get feedback to make sure you understood the point of the conversation.

Some couples find it helpful to take turns in the speaker and listener roles to make sure both partners have the chance to be heard. If you do this, it can be helpful to use a prop to remind you who is in the speaker role at a given time. For example, some couples use a piece of tile because it signifies that the person holding it has "the floor." See *Couples' Corner* at the end of the book for an exercise that focuses on this skill.

Be Polite

One aspect of communication that is often neglected between people who know each other well is politeness. People often show more courtesy to strangers than they do to the people they love. However, being polite is more than just a social nicety. It is a way of demonstrating respect and honor for the person you love.

There are many ways you can express respect for your partner, and these approaches can have powerful positive effects on communication. First, communicating in a way that lets your partner know that you are a team helps keep the tone of a conversation positive. Second, showing a genuine interest in your partner's life and expressing affection in a variety of ways shows love and respect. Finally, being able to admit when you are wrong demonstrates that you are willing to look at the issues fairly and objectively.

Being polite is especially important when you have advice or criticism. Before giving advice or constructive criticism, you may want to think about whether it will be truly helpful to your partner, or whether it is really an indirect way of expressing feelings such as anger. If you find yourself talking about old history or dredging up issues from the past, you may be more interested in winning an argument than in providing helpful feedback.

What Are You Thinking?

Communication between partners takes place on many levels. People often read between the lines to try to understand the intent—as well as the literal meaning—of what somebody is saying. Although it is a natural process, misinterpretations can be the source of many communication problems for a couple. The interpretations of the things others say are often strongly influenced by personal thoughts and feelings. As a result, intentions can easily be misunderstood, leading to potentially serious communication problems.

Sometimes our own thoughts can lead us to misinterpret a situation. These incorrect or distorted thoughts are called *cognitive distortions*. Often such cognitive distortions arise from strongly held beliefs that we have about ourselves, which may have developed in childhood. Many people become so used to filtering the world through these distortions that the process becomes automatic. As a result, it can take a great deal of effort to recognize that these distortions exist, and even more effort to correct them. In the next few pages, we'll discuss some common cognitive distortions and provide examples of how they might affect the way couples communicate.

Mind Reading

It is natural for people to assume they know all there is to know about their partner's feelings and the motives for their actions. But this belief can lead to some serious misunderstandings. Our assumptions about the motives of other people can be distorted by our own past experiences and current concerns. These distortions can lead to serious misinterpretations of another person's intent.

FRED HAS BEEN GIVING Bonnie hugs less often than he did before she began treatment for breast cancer. Bonnie notices the change in his behavior and assumes it is because he is no longer attracted to her. But he is actually avoiding giving her embraces because he is afraid he will cause her pain.

In this example, Bonnie made an incorrect assumption about why Fred was avoiding hugging her. This illustrates the importance of sharing your assumptions out loud with your partner. Having open and honest discussions gives your partner a chance to correct any misunderstandings before they cause problems in the relationship.

Tunnel Vision

Some people have such strong expectations of what their partner will say that they filter out any part of the message that doesn't fit with those expectations. This is sometimes referred to as *tunnel vision*. People with tunnel vision expect others to be hurtful or critical. As a result, they will usually find evidence to back up these expectations, even in messages that are intended to be supportive.

KEITH WAS DISTRESSED that Alicia was always busy running errands and working. He wanted to spend more time relaxing with her. One day at supper time, he said, "Hon, I worry about you working so hard. You do a great job with things but you are always running around doing everything, and we never have any time to talk or be together. I appreciate everything you're doing, but sometimes I just wish you would slow down and stop trying to be a superwoman."

Alicia blew up. "You have some nerve telling me to slow down when I'm doing everything around here! You don't have the right to criticize me when I'm doing it all, without any help from you."

In this example, Alicia completely misses Keith's main points: she is doing a good job, he appreciates all her hard work, and he misses spending quality time with her.

Magnification

With *magnification*, a small slight or hurt becomes exaggerated to the point where it seems like a catastrophe. It is often apparent in the words a person uses to describe a situation. Words that represent extremes like "awful," "always," or "never" are usually red flags for magnification.

ONE MORNING, YVONNE AND BOB were having breakfast. Yvonne looked at Bob and said, "Honey, you look a little tired today."

Later that day, Yvonne overheard Bob talking on the phone to a friend. "Yvonne thinks I look like death. She always says I look tired no matter how energetic I act or feel."

All or None Thinking

Some people tend to view people and situations in an all-or-nothing way. They tend to see things as right or wrong, good or bad, healthy or unhealthy. People who have *all or none* thinking often have a lot of trouble seeing a situation from a different perspective than their own. They also often have a hard time accepting compromises that partially meet each partner's needs. Another common result of this type of thinking is that it can cause people to idealize their partners at one moment and be critical of them the next.

Although Yvonne always accompanied Bob to his doctor's appointments, she asked Bob to go alone one day because she felt she had too much to do at home. Afterwards, when she had a moment to think about it, she felt terribly guilty about not taking Bob. She felt she had let him down as a wife and had failed to support him in his time of need. But in truth, Bob was fine with going by himself, and had in fact wondered in the past if she wouldn't prefer to sometimes stay home and catch up on things when he had appointments.

Global Labeling

Global labeling occurs when other people, behaviors, or events are summed up in one word. Global labels, such as "cheap," "lazy," or "greedy," are inaccurate labels for two reasons: first, to sum up a person, action, or event in one word treats it as if there are no other qualities worth considering. This is especially hurtful when it is directed at a person. Second, global labels usually do not apply to all situations. For instance, people may seem lazy if they are not motivated but may work hard at something they find important or interesting.

The use of global labels can have a chilling effect on communication between partners. Partners who are labeled typically react defensively because they view the label as critical and unfair.

Sometimes Fred leaves his dirty clothes lying around. This happens more often now that Bonnie has started her treatments, and Fred has more to do around the house. But Bonnie gets exasperated, telling Fred, "You're a slob who will never change! You've never been this messy before!"

Fractured Logic

Fractured logic occurs when people base their thinking on a general conclusion about one or two small events. With fractured logic, someone's interpretation of a situation goes so far beyond what actually occurred, he or she inevitably comes to the wrong conclusion. As happens with most cognitive distortions, the conclusion often has much more to do with a person's own feelings and concerns than with the reality of the situation.

> KEITH THINKS TO HIMSELF, "Alicia's been late coming home the past two nights. I don't think she wants to come home at all."

Control Fallacies

People who have *control fallacies* feel either completely responsible for their relationship problems or believe that everything is completely out of their control. Either of these extremes can be frustrating for the person experiencing the distorted thinking and his or her partner.

> ALICIA KNOWS THAT SHE CAN'T CONTROL that her husband has leukemia. However, she's sure if she puts her mind to it, she can get Keith to agree to every type of treatment his doctor recommends. In truth, though, Keith is more inclined to be selective about which treatments he undergoes. He doesn't want to receive any treatments that are highly risky or experimental or that reduce his quality of life.

The reality of the situation is that Alicia cannot *make* Keith behave differently. What she can do is express to Keith her fear that he won't recover if he doesn't undergo every available treatment. She can also ask Keith to discuss his treatment plan with her before making any decisions.

Express Your Feelings

Even for people in intimate, supportive relationships, talking about feelings can be problematic. However, being open and honest with your partner about both positive and negative feelings will strengthen your relationship. There are several things you can do to make discussing feelings easier and more helpful to the relationship.

When you are talking about your feelings, try to be as specific as possible. For example, to say that you are "upset" can mean a variety of things, from

How to Deal with Cognitive Distortions

Some people, such as those who suffer from depression, are particularly likely to experience cognitive distortions; however, everyone interprets relationship situations incorrectly from time to time. Below are several questions you can ask yourself to guard against cognitive distortions and correct misconceptions in your thinking:

❥ What evidence do I have to support my interpretation of the situation?

❥ What evidence goes against my interpretation?

❥ Are there any other explanations for my partner's behavior that I haven't considered?

❥ Have I leapt to a conclusion without knowing all the facts?

Most importantly, though, you can discuss any concerns you have with your partner. This gives you both a chance to clear the air and correct any mistaken conclusions that either of you may have reached.

worried to sad. Because certain words can have more than one meaning, the chances that your partner will misunderstand what you are saying increase. But if you say, "I feel hurt" or "I feel angry" instead, the meaning is much clearer. You can state your feelings even more clearly by using modifying words. For example, saying "I am really angry" has a different impact than saying, "I am angry." Adding other details, such as how long you have felt a certain way and what made you feel that way, can help your partner understand your feelings even better.

If you feel upset because of something your partner has done, it helps to put your feelings in context. You may realize your feelings are much stronger than seems reasonable given the situation. This may be because something in your family history causes you to be especially sensitive to certain situations. Or you may already be irritated by something else that happened that day. Regardless of what is contributing to the intensity of the feelings you experience, letting your partner know this information can help him or her to better understand your response. It will help your partner respond less defensively, and it also increases the chances you will get a response that is caring and supportive.

Body language is another way people express feelings. While people are talking, they also communicate with gestures and tone of voice. Sincerity comes across when behavior and words match. But sometimes people develop habits that result in mixed messages. For example, some people laugh when they are anxious or sad, and some people cross their arms or avoid eye contact when their partner is talking. Actions can sometimes speak louder than words, so it is useful to pay attention to body language and tone of voice when talking to other people, particularly a significant other.

Up to this point, we have been focusing on communicating negative feelings. However, some people have as much or more difficulty expressing positive feelings as they do expressing negative ones. Even if you are sure that your partner knows how much you love, admire, or appreciate him or her, it never hurts to say it.

Ask for What You Need

Many people have problems asking other people for things they need. In relationships, this often results in one or both partners feeling resentful. People assume that their partner already knows what they want and just doesn't care enough to provide it. It can be remarkably effective for people to ask for what they need rather than let resentment build.

Before asking for what you want or need from your partner, first try to think about exactly what you would like him or her to do. The more precise you are, the easier it will be for your partner to respond in the way you prefer. Try to focus your request only on specific behaviors that you would like changed. For example, you might ask, "Can you please pick up your dirty clothes?" instead of saying, "Don't be a slob." Your partner is only able to control his or her actions. Any attempt to change someone's personality, values, attitudes, or feelings is not only likely to fail, but it is also likely to cause a defensive reaction. When you are making a request, it can also help to talk about how the situation makes you feel, such as, "I feel overwhelmed when I see so many things that need to be done around the house."

No matter how nicely you ask for something from your partner, there is no guarantee that he or she will agree to your request. With the many demands that cancer places on a couple's time, energy, and other resources, each partner may be unable to meet the needs of the other completely, no matter how much they would like to. When this situation arises, rather than blaming a "stubborn" partner, it helps to work together to reach a compromise that at least partially meets both of your needs.

Ways to Resolve Conflicts

Even with the best efforts to express feelings and needs appropriately, conflict is inevitable in any relationship. During stressful times, conflict is especially likely to occur.

In any conflict, the way you initially approach the issue is critical to the outcome—it sets the tone for the entire discussion. When you first present your side of the issue, it is best to express yourself as gently and diplomatically as possible. The expression, "You can catch more flies with honey than with vinegar," applies perfectly to this situation. People naturally respond more favorably when they are addressed respectfully. Also, it helps to frame your statements as "I" statements rather than "you" statements.

Discussions usually end on the same note that they began. If you begin a conversation with criticism, sarcasm, defensiveness, or contempt, the chances are that your partner will adopt the same tone. However, it is never too late to try to bring things back on the right track. If a conflict begins more harshly than you intended or you find yourself in the middle of a defensive response, there are things that you can say to help bring a more respectful tone to the conversation. Some statements that can help soften the tone of an argument include the following:

- I'm scared.
- Did I do something wrong?
- That hurt my feelings.
- I don't feel like you understand me right now.
- I need your support right now.
- Can we take a break?
- I blew it. Can we start over?
- I'm sorry. Please forgive me.

- Let's try to find some common ground.
- I could be wrong here.
- We are getting off track.
- I understand.
- I know this isn't your fault.
- I see what you're saying.

If a conflict ever progresses to the point that you feel your emotions are too intense to listen closely to your partner's perspective or to keep the conversation respectful, it may be time to walk away and take a break. The break should last at least twenty minutes to allow your body and mind time to calm down. It may help to take extra steps to soothe yourself during this time by doing such things as breathing deeply, relaxing your muscles, listening to relaxing music, or talking a brief walk outside. After a break that gives each partner a chance to cool down, it is often much easier to come to an acceptable solution to the conflict.

Compromise Is Key

Compromise is necessary in any relationship, but the demands of a major illness make it essential. If partners insist on getting their way, one person will win, one person will lose, and the relationship will suffer.

WHILE BONNIE WAS UNDERGOING TREATMENT, she felt too fatigued to do her usual household chores. Although he wasn't used to it, Fred began cleaning the house and doing the laundry. Fred was too proud to ask for help or instructions, so he washed light and dark clothes together and used the wrong cleansers on the stove.

Bonnie soon found herself criticizing Fred for the way he was doing the housework. He became irritated at Bonnie's constant criticism because he felt unappreciated for trying to help out. After a heated argument, Bonnie and Fred realized that they could make a compromise. Fred could do the chores without unwanted advice or criticism from Bonnie as long as she could teach him the basic rules of cleaning and laundering.

In any conflict, it is worthwhile to consider ways to reach a compromise. One way to work out a compromise is to develop a partnership contract. Like any other type of contract, a partnership contract states what is expected from each partner. Partners can bargain for the things they value most, while giving their partner something that they value. Some couples write and sign their contracts as an indication of their honest intent to follow through with the agreement. This process can help the couple feel like they reached a fair solution to their conflict. It also can take some of the emotional heat out of sensitive discussions.

Steps to Problem Solving

Some issues between partners simply need to be discussed so that each person understands the other's position. Other problems, however, need to be actively solved. If you have fully discussed an issue but the conflict continues, you may need to shift your attention to active problem solving.

There are four basic steps to solving any problem:
1. Define the problem.
2. Think of a possible solution.
3. Agree on the best course of action.
4. Act on the mutually agreed upon solution.

Although these steps make problem solving seem easy, each step presents its own challenges. Sometimes it is extremely difficult to define the problem. People may think one thing is the problem, when it is actually another. For example, Bruce thinks his wife is too focused on the children. In reality, though, the problem is that they are not intimate enough as a couple. If she were to focus less on the children, Bruce may still not be satisfied because he is not getting what he wants out of the relationship. If a couple can agree on the real problem, then they may be able to resolve it together.

Finding solutions to a problem can also be challenging. If you find your-self having problems coming up with potential solutions, brainstorming may help. The idea behind brainstorming is simply to throw out ideas without worrying about how good those ideas are. Neither partner should criticize these ideas as they are suggested. Once you have multiple possible solutions on the table, you and your partner can choose among many options instead of arguing in favor of one or two. With many possible solutions, you may even be able to combine some in a way that helps each partner feel successful.

Once you have agreed on a possible solution to the problem, you can test your solution over a trial period. Following that period, each partner can then comment on how the solution seems to be working. If necessary, you may need to make some changes or look for completely different solutions.

Core Arguments

We first discussed core arguments in Chapter 5. These are arguments that seem to keep coming back in different ways throughout the relationship. They usually relate to basic issues like trust, security, and power.

The strategies for dealing with conflict that we have been discussing, such as on pages 139–140, also work to resolve core argumnets. Because core arguments relate to basic values, it is more difficult to resolve them by compromise. It may require more discussion over time to come to a solution that is acceptable to each partner. You may even find that no matter how much work you put into discussing the issue, you and your partner will not see eye to eye.

If you can't agree on how to settle a core argument, you can still limit the damage it does to your relationship. If you are able to discuss your differences calmly and respectfully, you can gain a genuine appreciation of where your partner is coming from. Even if you do not agree with his or her position, accepting your partner's position will allow you to move on from the core argument and enjoy the other aspects of your relationship.

Take Personal Responsibility for Your Needs

If you come to the point where you realize that you and your partner are unable to reach an agreement on something that you feel strongly about, it may be necessary to accept personal responsibility to take care of it for yourself. Even at the best of times, no partner can give you everything you desire. When someone has been diagnosed with cancer, they have even more competing demands that can prevent them from meeting your needs. Although it can be painful to realize this, you have the power to take care of your own needs.

Practical Tips for Improving Communication

This chapter has provided several suggestions on how to improve communication and resolve conflicts more effectively. Like learning any other skill, improving your communication takes practice and effort. The following activities and tips are designed to help you start this learning process. See the workbook (*Couples' Corner*) at the end of this book for more structured exercises.

➤ Learning to listen well is perhaps the most important step in improving communication. Try this exercise to practice active listening. Think of a situation when you didn't think your partner understood your perspective. Then try to present the issue again for your partner. After you have given your side of the story, have your partner repeat it to you in different words. If your partner didn't get the correct message, keep trying until he or she can finally present your side of the issue accurately.

➤ Start slowly. Discussions about truly important issues—no matter what they may be—are always difficult, so don't rush. You may have a hard time finding the right words to describe feelings, but keep trying until you are able to express how you feel.

➤ Listen to what is said. If you aren't clear about what your partner means, ask for clarification. Don't guess or assume what something means.

➤ Be honest. Understand that being honest does not mean being blunt, tactless, or unkind. It means discussing real and projected events and sharing emotional reactions to those events. Don't pretend that you're not concerned or afraid or angry if you are.

➤ Talking about death can be hard for everyone. However, it will not only help your partner understand your feelings, but it will also give you a chance to talk about how much you mean to each other.

➤ If it seems useful, seek help from a trusted person outside the family to guide conversations that are difficult for you. If you are not making progress in improving communication in your relationship on your own, consider getting help from a couples therapist or counselor.

Taking steps to meet your own needs when your partner is unable or unwilling to do so can take some pressure off your partner, as well as improve your overall satisfaction with the relationship. For example, if you would like to get out of the house more often, but your partner is rarely interested, go out with other people who enjoy the same activities that you do. If your partner does not give you enough appreciation and support, try building new friendships. Or if you would like more meals at home, try cooking them for yourself.

Improving communication in a relationship can be hard work. However, this effort can also be rewarding. Good communication is crucial for solving problems that you face as a couple and for building intimacy. In the next chapter, we will take a closer look at ways to create a greater sense of emotional closeness and connection as a couple.

Chapter Nine

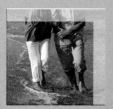

Creating
Emotional Intimacy

The stressful experience of cancer can create distance between intimate partners, even when they were previously very close. The fears that cancer can bring, as well as the disruption in your lives and the physical discomfort of treatment, can interfere with the closeness and openness that you may have had with your partner before the cancer diagnosis.

In this chapter, we will look at ways to maintain and enhance emotional closeness with your partner both during and after cancer treatment. We will talk about how greater self-knowledge and self-acceptance can enhance intimacy. We will also explore shared activities that promote closeness and look at the importance of rebuilding your teamwork and cooperation.

Developing Intimacy through Self-Acceptance

To be intimate with someone, you need to be comfortable enough with who you are, so you can be spontaneous and open with each other. Fully knowing and accepting yourself—your likes and dislikes, strengths and weaknesses, mistakes and successes, and every aspect of your history—will enhance your close relationships.

There is also a sense of balance in a relationship when both partners are content with who they are and know how to find the things that nourish them in life. This is, of course, an ideal, and most people feel dissatisfied with some aspects of their lives. Nonetheless, it is helpful to hold in your mind the image of this ideal as one that you can begin to work towards. Even small increases in your ability to be comfortable being yourself can make a big difference in how close you feel to others—and how close they feel to you.

Being in a satisfying close relationship can also help you accept yourself, and this can become a positive cycle. It is a rare and special relationship in which the growth of the relationship goes hand in hand with your own growth as an individual. In such relationships, people typically feel energetic and alive. And growth in yourself and in your relationship is nourishing, not draining. So we emphasize that ideal relationships are those in which you accept yourself *and* each other, and these feelings are strengthened as the relationship grows (see Chapter 4 for more characteristics of a good relationship).

On the flip side, a draining relationship is one in which your experiences in the relationship sap your self-esteem. One woman who had struggled throughout her nineteen-year marriage with an excessively critical spouse tearfully stated, "I feel like I'm half the person I used to be." Her own self-perception suffered as a result of her experiences in the relationship. A negative cycle may develop when your self-esteem is low, and you are in a draining or even abusive relationship. Getting out of the bad situation can be a way to start mending your sense of self as an individual.

To strengthen your sense of self, invest some time by pursuing interests that are meaningful to you as an individual, separate from your partner. This will help you define yourself—both as an individual and as a member of a couple. If you feel uncomfortable with aloneness or independence from your partner, see if you can gradually increase your comfort level. Some feelings of dependence are a normal and expected part of being attached to somebody, but consult with a professional therapist if you feel overly dependent. If you have developed the idea that your partner has to be there to take care of everything for you, your self-esteem has likely suffered as a consequence.

Some people find themselves waiting for a rescue to come—as if by magic—from their persistent life struggles. To some degree, these "rescue fantasies" are a universal part of human existence. Nonetheless, fantasy needs to

The Path to Self-Acceptance

How do you strengthen your sense of self and be part of a couple? Here are some tips for you to consider:

- Do not define yourself through another person. We all need and want relationships, but other people cannot tell us who we are. We must find that out for ourselves.

- You can get to know yourself by spending time with yourself. That means you must spend time alone.

- Rather than focusing on the relationship, focus on your identity as an individual. Value yourself as an individual, and not just as part of a couple.

- If you are waiting for someone to do something for you that you don't want to do for yourself, stop. Do what needs to be done, and in the process empower yourself.

- Learn to be alone and be comfortable with it.

- Take responsibility for your own struggles. Stand up for yourself.

- Say nice things to yourself about yourself.

be separated from reality. To start with, it often helps to define the problems by asking, "What is it exactly that I am waiting for my life partner to do for me?" Next, ask yourself whether your fantasy outcome is realistic. If not, define a realistic end goal, and see if you can identify a sequence of steps you can take, one by one, towards achieving it. If you can identify an end goal but get hopelessly stuck on the steps, ask a friend for perspective, or consider consulting with a professional.

Investing in yourself also means standing up for yourself. Are there situations in which you'd like to stand up for yourself more? Do you know how to do this? If not, get input from someone you trust.

If self-acceptance is a problem for you, start looking for things to compliment yourself on each day. If you tend to dwell on things you didn't do or think that you did wrong, it is often helpful to make a list at the end of the day of things you did do that deserve credit. The list should include not only productive activities, but also the "human" things like being nice to somebody you saw that day. Pay attention even to what you consider to be small accomplishments.

Developing Intimacy through Honesty

When you become comfortable with yourself, you can share more of your feelings with your loved ones. Being honest with your partner means being in touch with your own feelings and expressing them freely. Why is it necessary to be honest? Sharing what you truly feel is a way of becoming closer. When you decide to share who you are with your partner, you talk about your likes, dislikes, opinions, fears, and hopes. Even sharing events from your day-to-day life is a good way of expressing yourself. If your feelings are hurt, letting your partner know immediately can save both of you time and pain later. If your relationship has been distant for some time, or you are not used to expressing your feelings openly, consider whether you have been focused on expressing yourself such that you forget to ask your partner how he or she feels. Remember to take time to let your partner talk too (and encourage him or her to do so).

A cancer diagnosis can cause strong negative feelings such as disbelief, shock, fear, and anger. Many people are deeply worried about the anticipated disruption in their lives and the possibility of dying. You may feel you need to hide or minimize your feelings during this difficult time in order to protect your partner. But part of the process of being completely honest is facing the truth together about how you feel about the cancer. Avoiding the issue will only make the fear grow stronger. The best thing you can do for each other is to be honest about what you are feeling. It is okay to pace yourself if discussing these feelings gets overwhelming at first. Tell your partner if you feel the need to take a break and return to the conversation later.

Identify Your Feelings

Sometimes we have trouble identifying what it is that we are upset about. It can be helpful to ask yourself these questions:

❧ What am I afraid of?

❧ What is frustrating me?

❧ What is hurting me and why?

❧ When did I first notice this feeling?

❧ What was going through my mind when I got scared or upset?

Fears about the future and feelings of guilt, frustration, and confusion are often less frightening when you share them with your partner honestly and sensitively. Doing so can also help both of you feel free from the burden of unspoken fears and concerns that cancer has brought on. You can begin to build hope for the future together.

BONNIE HAS COMPLETED HER MONTHS OF TREATMENT for breast cancer. She is returning to her job as a real estate agent. Her office is about a thirty-minute drive from her home. She is eager to get out of the house because Fred is driving her crazy. As soon as she walks into another room and is quiet for a while, he anxiously calls out, "Are you OK?" "Yes, Fred—I'm fine." She is starting to lose patience. She has not said much about this to him, though, because she understands how anxious Fred feels about her health.

On her first day back at work, Bonnie discovers that Fred has been making excuses to call and leave messages for her so he can ask the secretary how she is doing. That evening, she sat Fred down and explained to him how she felt about his constant surveillance. It was unnecessary and made her feel more anxious. She confronted Fred about his anxiety for her safety and health. For the first time, they discussed what would happen if cancer did ultimately claim her life. Fred cried and told her that he just couldn't make it without her. Although this was painful for Bonnie to hear, she was able to point out Fred's strengths and make him promise not to do anything to hurt himself in the event she died. She encouraged him to seek counseling, which Fred is considering. But he already feels better because they have talked about the one issue they have been avoiding for months.

Ghosts from the Past

We have been looking at how knowing yourself and accepting who you are can help you achieve a deeper and more comfortable closeness with significant others. Understanding both yourself and your partner better often involves an exploration of your history and how it is reflected in your current style of interacting with one another. As we discussed in Chapter 2, our early experiences often influence how we experience relationships as adults. The manner in which our early experiences reappear in adult life is often subtle and may take us by surprise. It can feel as though you are living with ghosts from your past, some of whom may be actual people, such as parents (living or deceased) that continue to be present in your mind and heart even when physically absent. Other ghosts are experiences or "ways of being" in relationships that were typical of your upbringing or of your personal history.

Many of us look to our partners for nurturing, much like a parent. This is common and normal. For some people who were particularly disappointed by an actual parent, this longing may be stronger than average or even dominate their behavior in the current relationship. Other people may enter a relationship with the expectation that their current partner will replace a lost love from the past.

Some people may find themselves re-experiencing their early disappointments in their present relationships. This may happen for two reasons. First, we may *feel* as though history is repeating itself because we are quick to interpret events in the present based on our early experiences. For example, we may compare the times when we are disappointed in ways that are familiar from past experiences, while ignoring those instances when a loved one's behavior *doesn't* fit old patterns. Second, some people become comfortable with the sort of person who disappoints them, and it doesn't occur to them to look for a different type of mate. That being said, it bears repeating that your history isn't fate carved in stone, and everyone doesn't always automatically select partners who are just like their parents or other ghosts from the past.

If past relationships (especially with parents) are going to resurface, it will typically occur with those we feel closest to, especially in love relationships. In times of stress, we may be likely to fall back into habits learned at a young age. It is not surprising, then, that dealing with cancer can awaken ghosts from the past.

More specifically, the way that you respond to having cancer or having a partner with cancer may be similar to the way that people in your early life tended to respond to an illness. For example, if your parents usually ignored your physical complaints when you were growing up, you may find yourself ignoring your partner's complaints. It is often helpful to talk with each other about how your early experiences may have influenced your current behavior and how these experiences were different for the two of you. Then you can begin to help each other to learn ways of responding to one another that each of you finds most comforting.

Nurturing Your Love

Another central part of creating satisfying, intimate relationships is expressing positive feelings and affection. It may be hard to come up with positive thoughts or feelings if you are under a great deal of stress or have been frustrated or angry with your partner. It is sometimes easier to focus on the negative aspects of relationships than the positives. It is somewhat like the "no news is good news" scenario. If our partners do what we expect, we say nothing. When they step over the line, we are the first to call it to their attention.

Heightening your awareness of each other's positive contributions is one good way to change these negative patterns and nurture intimacy with your partner. Allow yourself to explore all aspects of your partner as a person. He or she may have skills or talents that you admire, even everyday skills such as fixing things around the house. There may be things about your partner's body, face, or touch that you find especially pleasing. It may be as simple as thinking about more carefree times you've had with your partner, before the cancer diagnosis.

Although these kinds of thought exercises may seem contrived or forced, there is evidence that if you are able to shift the focus of your thoughts towards some positive aspects of your relationship, your emotional responses may follow. This isn't a replacement for addressing problematic aspects of the relationship, but it can be a good place to start.

Thinking positively about your shared ventures and the things that you have created as a couple can also be helpful during this stressful time. For some couples, this may be your children, or your household, the "safe haven" you have created together. Other couples have a shared passion for an activity, such as music. There may be something that you accomplish well as a team, such as parenting or a mutual hobby.

In addition to thinking positively about your relationship and nurturing your feelings of affection for your partner, expressing these feelings is just as important. This involves doing or saying things that please your partner. Just like redirecting your thoughts, it can feel unnatural to try doing something positive if you aren't feeling that way. But doing positive things for your partner even when you don't feel that positive can be a way of getting the ball rolling. We suggest you try a small positive behavior first and see how it feels. Chances are you'll like the results.

Examples of positive behaviors that please your partner can include helping out at home, offering a special activity or meal, paying your partner a compliment, or simply expressing your love in words or with an affectionate touch. If you are unsure of what your partner would enjoy, offer some choices. For example, you might say, "I'd like to do something for you tonight. Would you like it if I cooked dinner, or if I gave you a back rub?" Asking your partner questions about his or her feelings, and listening well, is another example of a pleasing behavior. If you begin engaging in pleasing behavior, your partner's behavior will follow, which begins a positive cycle in the relationship. If your relationship has become boring, irritating, or otherwise unsatisfying, mutual expressions of good will can be a great place to start improving things.

Ways to Share

After a diagnosis of cancer, a couple may become increasingly busy and pre-occupied with all of the things that suddenly need to be done that they lose touch with each other—and yet this is the time when it is most critical to work together. Here are some suggestions for activities that could help you to reconnect with your partner:

- Spend some time together researching the illness and the best ways to treat it.

- Make a list of all of the things you need to do to support each other throughout this process.

- Practice relaxation exercises together.

- Listen to music together.

- Play cards or a board game.

- Go for short walks together.

- Work in the garden together.

- Put together a scrapbook or photo album while talking and sharing special memories.

- Develop new family rituals.

- Appreciate and acknowledge the things that you do for each other.

- Check in with each other at the end of the day to see how each of you is feeling and what you can do to help each other.

Work Less, Play More

Becoming comfortable being yourself can be a way of becoming closer to your partner. There are certain settings where we feel completely comfortable being ourselves, and it is in these places that we feel peace and contentment. For many of us, this is not true in everyday life, so we have to make time for play.

How do we "play" as adults? One important part of play is surrendering our adult attitudes and responsibilities, even for a short time. Playing as an adult implies a sense of freedom. For some people, playing may be spending a rainy day indoors reading. For others, playing would be taking a long trek through the woods. The main thing is to have fun, feel free, and do what you enjoy.

YVONNE AND BOB WERE NEVER VERY PLAYFUL before the cancer came along; they were both involved with their respective careers. When they met Ted and Carol, who had also been through cancer, they began getting together for dinner. Soon they found some card games and board games that all enjoyed. They looked forward to being silly and laughing for the entire evening. Now they consider that part of their life a necessity to keep them from falling into despair over the cancer situation. One night Bob didn't feel well enough to play. Instead, he watched and enjoyed laughing with them as they played. They are determined to keep the laughter coming in the months ahead.

Building Closeness through Spiritual Exploration

Discovering who you are and understanding yourself is a necessary step towards being close with your significant other. For many people, this includes awareness of a spiritual side. Spirituality, in the broadest sense, may be organized religion, exploration of the meaning of existence, activities that help us see a larger purpose in our experiences, or activities that strengthen our moral values. The good feeling that comes with connection to the larger universe or to a spiritual or moral framework can help you develop self-esteem and improve your capacity to be close to others.

Many faiths hold certain values as a gold standard of behavior. Whether learned within a religious congregation, a community of faith, or in any other setting, principles such as being loving, kind, honest, and patient can offer a helpful standard for behavior that serves us well in all situations in life, including relationships. As you put your own chosen principles into practice, people are likely to reward you with like behavior in return. Ultimately, having such a framework and working towards meeting your personal ideals for behavior can help you to be more satisfied with your life and relationships.

Many religious, existential, or moral perspectives can also help you see the big picture, allowing you to stop dwelling on your own or others' past mistakes, thereby enhancing both self-acceptance and forgiveness. For example, a smoker with lung cancer can experience painful self-blame on a daily basis. It can lead to tremendous healing if a broader spiritual or existential perspective allows the person's partner to say, "I don't blame you for smoking cigarettes and getting cancer. I have done things in my life that are unhealthy too. I don't think you deserve punishment. Let's just move past all of that and focus on today, and how you and I are going to deal with this." As one pastor once stated, "Believing in something bigger than yourself often brings people help, hope, and a home."

Finally, if you are a member of a religious community or any other larger social group, these communities can often provide the type of support that a couple dealing with cancer may need. Churches, synagogues, and other religious and social organizations can support couples in crisis with concrete needs like food and transportation, but also with that all-important morale boost.

Finding Common Ground and Working As a Team

If cancer has changed or disrupted your relationship, you may need to find common ground where both of you can feel relaxed together again. If connecting in a sexual or more intimate way seems difficult, try first to connect as friends who share common interests and just have fun together. Focus on the things that both of you enjoy doing or talking about. Spending time just doing relaxing and stress-free things together will allow you both to recover and lay the groundwork for reconnecting emotionally. In the next chapter, we will talk more specifically about sexual intimacy, and help you find ways to strengthen this part of your relationship during and after cancer.

When both of you are recovering from a stressful experience and the relationship seems to have suffered as a consequence, working as a team will be fundamental to your healing. One sign that teamwork has broken down is an intense focus on the other's apparent faults or shortcomings. Focusing on someone else's imperfections can be a way of avoiding your own responsibility for the problems between you, or it can be a way of feeling better about yourself by seeing your partner as inferior. Regardless of why the teamwork has broken down, try to shift your focus towards a more balanced view of one another that includes strengths as well as weaknesses. Another sign of a breakdown in your teamwork is an exclusive focus on winning arguments rather than working towards a more constructive and mutually positive outcome. Of course, when you stop trying to win the fight, you also will find that you are more forgiving of the other person's shortcomings.

In the spirit of teamwork, there are several destructive patterns to avoid. If you plan to work towards healing in your relationship, it is crucial to avoid making any threats to leave the relationship. Even at your most angry or distressed moment, resist the temptation to pull the "I'm getting a divorce" card. Threatening your partner obviously works against the goals of healing and cooperation.

If you know you want the best for your relationship, make sure that you are back in the business of working towards that. By having higher expectations, you show respect and honor for both your present and future relationship. If being close has become the same thing as treating each other like enemies, you may need to play act first, treating each other as you would treat guests at your house—in order to restore a respectful environment. The bottom line is that teamwork and a constructive atmosphere are crucial to healing your relationship both during and after an exhausting encounter with cancer.

Removing Obstacles

There are a number of behaviors that can interfere with closeness simply by keeping you physically apart and distracted by other activities and relationships. Examples include developing new intimate friendships that replace time spent with your partner, beginning a demanding side business, or having a packed schedule that takes you outside the house for much of the week.

Practical Tips for Creating Intimacy

This chapter has provided you with some suggestions to help foster intimacy. Creating closeness, connection, and emotional intimacy takes practice. The following activities are designed to help you develop these skills. They provide a safe way of getting to know yourself and each other better. See the workbook (*Couples' Corner*) at the end of this book for more structured exercises.

- Give each other positive feedback about the relationship. It is all too easy to allow the difficulties to outweigh the strengths, especially when you are upset.

- Make a list of things that you like about your partner. These could include qualities such as his or her energy, intelligence, passion, wit, gentleness, skill as a parent, ability to understand you, or capacity to make you feel safe or comforted.

- Make an effort to remember the things that you have always appreciated in your partner, and the reasons that you were drawn to each other in the first place. These positive feelings can protect both of you from stress. Share them with one another.

- You may have never come to know every aspect of your partner. Try thinking about him or her as a mysterious person or as a stranger. Ask questions about how he or she feels about things other than the cancer. What does your partner consider to be his or her most painful experiences? What was the happiest time in your partner's life? What are some things that your partner knows about you that no one else knows?

Whether these behaviors occur because you want to avoid the problems between you and your partner or because of practical issues, they need to be addressed to rebuild closeness. You need to find a way to put some of that energy back into the relationship to be fully intimate again.

This doesn't mean that you have to give up all sports, hobbies, or outside friendships. Many of these pursuits meet basic needs. But both of you may need to prioritize which activities are essential, and which you can be flexible in letting go. It is also worth asking yourself, "Am I doing this activity to avoid spending time with my spouse?" If the answer is yes, you will need to identify the problems you might be avoiding and make a decision about how to address them.

Chapter Ten

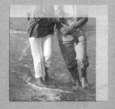

Strengthening
Physical Intimacy

A good sexual relationship is a natural outgrowth of the emotional intimacy you have nurtured as a couple. Trust is an essential part of a satisfying sex life. If you are unable to trust your partner in some way, this can lead to difficulty relaxing and responding to one another during sex. Fully accepting each other is also necessary to be completely sexually responsive as a couple. If one or both of you is preoccupied with the other's flaws, this may lead to an environment in which it is not possible to be open enough for sex. If this is the case, it may be necessary to address the difficulty with the help of a professional therapist before working on your sexual intimacy (see Chapter 12 for more information about professional services).

It also helps to spend time together outside the bedroom. If you have not spent time with each other all day, then expecting sexual ecstasy in the evening may not be realistic. The bottom line is that when both of you feel completely safe emotionally, close to each other, and free to be yourselves with one another, your sexual relationship will likely be more creative and energetic. Make sure that you are not substituting sexual activity for closeness. A satisfying relationship requires closeness both inside and outside the bedroom.

Although sex is a basic part of life, doctors and patients often don't talk about the effects of cancer treatment on sexuality. There are several things to keep in mind regarding sex when being treated for cancer. This chapter explores ways to keep your sexual relationship strong during and after cancer treatment.

Be Informed and Communicate Clearly

The most important part of a good sexual relationship is good communication (see Chapter 8), and this may be especially true when someone has been diagnosed with cancer. Sex is one way for a couple to feel close. If you or your partner has been ill, depressed, or distant, you may fear that a sexual advance is too demanding. There are ways to bring up the topic of sex in a sensitive and assertive way. Avoid accusations such as, "You never touch me anymore!" Also avoid out-and-out demands such as, "We simply have to have sex soon. I can't stand the frustration!" Instead, try to express your feelings positively. You might say, "I really miss our sex life. Let's talk about what's getting in the way."

Communication with your health care team is also key. Talking honestly with your health care team can help you gain a better understanding of what you can and cannot do before, during, and after treatment. Be persistent, and don't stop asking until you get the information you want. If your doctor seems unresponsive to your questions, try a nurse or another member of your health care team. Learning as much as you can about the common effects of your cancer treatment on sexual functioning will help you and your partner adapt. The more you know about what sexual changes to expect, the better you can cope with these changes and resume a healthy sex life.

How to Cope with Changes in Appearance

All people tend to overestimate their physical imperfections when compared with others' judgments. What's more, after cancer treatment, it is normal to focus only on the part of the body that has been affected. For example, a woman who has had a mastectomy may be afraid of how her partner will feel seeing her unclothed.

If you or your partner seem uncomfortable with the changes in the other's body, it's best if you both talk openly about it. Sometimes such reactions reflect other problems in the relationship that need to be addressed and have nothing to do with changes in the patient's appearance. In other cases, the initial discomfort will be eased just by talking about it and will fade over time

Questions to Ask Your Health Care Team

Below is a list of suggested questions to ask your health care team about the effects of your treatment on your sexuality and what, if any, activities you should avoid during each phase of your treatment:

❥ How will this treatment (surgery, chemotherapy, radiation) affect my desire for sex?

❥ How will this treatment affect my ability to feel pleasure in my genital areas?

❥ How will this treatment affect my ability to reach an orgasm?

❥ Am I likely to have pain during sex as a result of this treatment?

❥ How will this treatment affect my ability to have an erection and ejaculate?

❥ Will this treatment cause me to go through menopause?

❥ Will it interfere with my taking an estrogen replacement after menopause?

❥ How will this treatment affect my ability to have children in the future?

❥ Will the effects be temporary or permanent?

❥ Will my appearance change?

❥ Is there any reason that I should *not* have sex while undergoing treatment?

Depending on the type of treatment you are receiving, there may be other problems you should be aware of that are not listed here. Be sure to discuss your particular concerns about sexual difficulties with your treatment team.

as both people adjust to the changes. It may be that the person who is uncomfortable just needs to find a way to openly express the feelings of fear and pain that have built up throughout the experience of dealing with cancer. Some people do not know how to cope with strong feelings except by withdrawing from all reminders of the painful feelings. Talk to a professional if this has happened to you.

Some physical changes caused by cancer treatment can be concealed. If you are just starting chemotherapy, you may want to shop for a head covering before your hair begins to fall out. Wigs can feel excessively warm and uncomfortable, so if you purchase one, you may decide to reserve it for certain occasions only. Many people feel a wig is too much trouble, especially since it is often hard to find one that looks natural. Alternatively, you can collect hats or scarves to wear during this phase of your treatment.

It's a good idea to discuss with your partner how each of you feels about wearing a wig or head covering during lovemaking. There is no right or wrong decision. Men often feel they should not be self-conscious about baldness resulting from treatment. Keep in mind, though, that losing hair during cancer treatment can be just as upsetting for men as for women.

How to Cope with an Imbalance in Desire

A common problem presented by couples with sexual difficulties is differences in sexual desire. This problem usually occurs later in the relationship, not in the beginning. The partner with stronger sexual interest may feel disappointed or personally wounded by the other's lack of desire. The partner with less desire may feel nagged or think that sex has become more important than his or her other qualities.

Both men and women often lose interest in sex during cancer treatment, at least for a time. This is quite normal. At first, concern for survival is so overwhelming that sex is far down on the list of needs to be met. Few people are interested in sex when they feel their lives are threatened. Other reasons for decreased desire can include pain or nausea, as well as emotional discomfort.

If you are the partner with cancer, your desire may be affected by anxiety about you or your partner's response to changes in your body. If this is the case, it is often helpful to talk about it until both of you feel comfortable enough to focus on being intimate. Although the focus may be on the cancer patient, even the healthy partner's desire for sex can be decreased by the stress of his or her partner's illness.

If all of the factors above have been addressed and your desire is still low, talk with your doctor. It also can be helpful to see if you can detect subtle changes in your desire. Everyone has a sexual thought or feeling from time to time, but we often ignore or forget them. If you have no interest in sex lately, try keeping a "Desire Diary." Prepare a sheet of paper for each day of the week, as shown in the example below. Take it with you wherever you go, keeping it somewhere secure and private. If you are worried about the paper being discovered, you can use shorthand that only you will be able to decipher. When you have a sexual thought or feeling, write it down. Note the time of day and whether you were alone or with someone. Also note what you did about the thought. Here is an example of one man's Desire Diary:

Monday			
Time	Who was with me?	Sexual thought or feeling	Action taken
7:30 A.M.	Wife	Wanted to caress my wife's breast while she was making breakfast.	None, because I knew she'd be annoyed.
1:30 P.M.	Alone	Noticed a good-looking woman by the coffee machine at work. Wondered what she'd look like without her clothes.	None.
3:15 P.M.	Alone	Thought about making love tonight	None.
10:00 P.M.	Wife	Felt turned-on when I got in bed	Asked her if she wanted to have sex. She said she was too tired, but maybe in the morning.

Although the writer of this diary did not have any sexual activity, he felt desire a few times during the day. Sometimes just keeping track of your desire will increase the number of sexual thoughts and feelings you notice. You might also find that certain settings or people help you feel more sexually responsive. Perhaps you think about sex most often in the morning or evening, or when you are at work, or in the presence of your partner. Once you have noted some patterns, you can arrange situations that spark a sexual mood.

Some people feel more sexually responsive if they get some exercise, plan a relaxed evening out with their partner, or make special efforts to look and feel sexy. Think about the things that have helped to get you into a sexy mood before. Try looking at erotic pictures, reading a sexy story, or watching a movie with a romantic or sexual plot. Fantasize about a sexual encounter, imagining it just as you would like it to be.

When you start feeling more sexually responsive by yourself, you can begin to share these feelings with your partner, and spend some time exploring them together.

How to Overcome Anxiety about Sex

Many couples believe sex should always happen on the spur of the moment, with little or no planning. If you feel awkward and nervous about trying some sexual touching, however, that perfect moment may never arrive. After an illness, many couples need to schedule relaxing time together and start their lovemaking slowly.

Part of the anxiety about resuming sex may be caused by the pressure to satisfy your partner. First, explore your own capacity to enjoy sex by using self-stimulation. Masturbation is not a necessary step in resuming your sex life, but it can be helpful. By touching yourself and even bringing yourself to orgasm, you can explore whether and in what ways cancer treatment has changed your sexual responses—without worrying about your partner's needs first.

If you feel uncomfortable with this approach, keep in mind that masturbation is a normal, natural behavior. Most men and women have tried touching their own genitals at some time in their lives, and those who enjoy good sex lives with their partners may still masturbate. Men and women in their seventies and eighties often still enjoy masturbating. Experience with masturbation often contributes to confidence when communicating about one's sexual responses with a partner.

If you feel at ease with the idea, try stroking more than just your genitals, but all the sensitive areas of your body. Notice the different feelings of pleasure

An Exercise to Help You Become Comfortable with Your Body Image

You may feel anxiety about resuming sex because you don't feel comfortable with your own body. What do you see when you look in the mirror? Many people notice only what they dislike about their looks—a pale complexion, hair loss, an ostomy appliance, or skinny legs. They fail to see an elegant profile, strong-looking hands, or a warm smile. The following mirror exercise can help you become more comfortable with the changes in your body:

❧ Find a time when you have at least fifteen minutes in private. Be sure to take enough time really to think about your appearance.

❧ Study yourself for the whole time, using the largest mirror you have. What parts of your body do you look at most? What do you avoid looking at? Can you catch yourself having critical thoughts about your body? What are your best features? Has cancer or its treatment changed the way you look?

❧ Try the mirror exercise when you look and feel good, such as before an evening out. If you normally wear clothing or accessories to disguise changes from cancer therapy, wear them during the mirror exercise. Practice this two or three times, or until you can look in the mirror and see at least three positive things about your looks.

❧ When you are comfortable seeing yourself as a stranger might see you, try the mirror exercise dressed as you would like to look for a lover. If you've had an ostomy, for example, wear a bathrobe that you like. Look at yourself for a few minutes, repeating the steps in the first mirror exercise. What is most attractive and sexy about you? Pay yourself at least three compliments on how you look.

❧ Finally, try the mirror exercise in the nude, without disguising any changes made by the cancer. If you have trouble looking at a scar, bare scalp, or an ostomy, take your time and allow yourself to get used to the area gradually. Most changes are not nearly as unattractive as they seem at first. If you feel tense while looking at yourself, take a deep breath and try to let all your muscles relax as you exhale. Don't stop the exercise until you have found three positive features—or, at the very least, remember the three compliments you paid yourself before.

The mirror exercise may also help you feel more relaxed when your partner looks at you. Ask your partner to tell you some of the things that are enjoyable about the way you look or feel physically. Explain that these positive views will help you feel better about yourself. Remember them when you are feeling unsure.

you can have. Later you can teach your partner any new discoveries you've made about your body's sensitive zones. Even if cancer treatment has not changed your sexual responses, you may invent some new caresses to enhance your sexual routine.

Resume Sexual Activity with Your Partner When You Feel Ready

After treatment, don't expect to "pick up where you left off" when it comes to sex. Schedule private time together, and make it relaxed, romantic, and special. Start the lovemaking slowly by gently touching each other's bodies, but not the genitals or breasts yet. Concentrate on the feelings of pleasure you are having. Many couples prefer to caress each other for a long while, gradually adding genital touching and building up the excitement over days or even weeks before resuming intercourse. And if intercourse is no longer possible or desired, you will still have learned much about bringing pleasure to yourself and your partner.

When you feel ready to try sexual touching with your partner, pick an occasion when you have time and privacy. You may want to set the scene to be especially relaxing. For example, you could light the room with candles or put on some soft music. Although you may feel a little shy, let your partner know as clearly and directly as you can that you would like to experiment with some sexual touching. You could even "make a date" to have some time alone together. You might say, "I feel ready for sex again, but I'd like to take things slowly. Would you be in the mood tonight to try a little touching? I can't promise it will go smoothly, but we can have fun trying."

It is a good idea for couples to put some limits on their touching the first few times they try sexual activity after cancer treatment. A good way to begin is with a special session devoted to all-over body touching. Each partner takes a turn touching and being touched. One partner lies face down on the bed, allowing the other partner to touch the entire back of the body, from toes to scalp. After about fifteen minutes, the partner lying down turns over so the front of the body can be touched. While being touched, your only job is to be self-centered and tune in to your own feelings. Don't worry about your partner's thoughts or feelings. When you are doing the touching, enjoy the shape and texture of your partner's body. Try many types of touching, varying light stroking and a firmer touch, as in a massage.

The first time you try a touching session, avoid the breasts and genitals. Your goals are to feel relaxed and to feel sensual pleasure. It is not essential to get sexually excited. If you agree on these goals before starting, the touching should not be frustrating or stressful. This type of session takes the nervousness and pressure out of being close again.

If you both feel relaxed during the first touching session, you can add some genital touching the next time. Over several sessions, partners can slowly spend more time on genital touching, until each one reaches an orgasm through stroking with a hand or through oral sex, if that is comfortable for both of you.

Be sure to take the time to relax and enjoy the time spent caressing and kissing each other. There should be no rush to complete the intercourse itself— that's the "dessert." Enjoy every course. This is a special time devoted to just you and your partner, doing something that you share together.

Many couples don't talk much about sex. After cancer treatment, however, your sexual routine may need to change. This calls for clear communication. This is not the time to let embarrassment silence you. Be sure to let your partner know, either in words or by guiding with your hand, the kinds of touches you like best. Try to express your desires in a positive way. For example, instead of saying, "Ouch! That's too rough!" you might say, "You have the right place, but I'd like you to use a light touch." Save intercourse until both partners really feel ready for it.

If cancer treatment has caused an inability to achieve an erection, inter-course may no longer be possible. Even though this is often felt as a great loss, couples can still enjoy all of the other parts of sex. It would be a shame to give up touching and caressing when there is no reason to.

One area of their marriage that had always been good for both Alicia and Keith was their sex life. They enjoyed sex, and seemed to have a well-matched level of sexual interest.

BETWEEN THE CANCER AND THE PHYSICAL AND EMOTIONAL TOLL of the treatment, not to mention all the other tasks they still had to keep up with, Keith and Alicia's sex life had totally died. They felt they were at an impasse. Keith had no interest in sex. He was bloated because of the chemotherapy, and he felt unattractive. He had no energy for sex and couldn't imagine how Alicia would still desire him.

Alicia felt it was really important to get this part of their relationship back. She began to talk with Keith about resuming some of their physical affection without it leading to sexual intercourse. They noticed that with hugging and kissing more often, they both felt closer to each other. They gradually began to think about having sex again.

One day, Alicia stopped her daily routine of household chores and lay with Keith in bed in the morning, after the kids were off playing with friends. They held each other and were quiet together. Before too much longer, they began making a "date" to have this intimate time. Sometimes they felt like having sex, but other times they just held each other and talked. Both of them felt rejuvenated by this renewed sexual relationship, which was different from before, yet very much alive.

Be Creative and Explore

No matter what kind of cancer treatment you or your partner has been through, you will almost always be able to be intimate and feel pleasure from touching. Most cancer treatments (other than those affecting some areas of the brain or spinal cord) do not damage the nerves and muscles involved in feeling pleasure from touch and reaching orgasm. Even men who cannot have erections or produce semen can still have the feeling of orgasm with the right kind of touching. Similarly, women with vaginal dryness can still achieve orgasm through touch.

Keep an open mind about ways to feel sexual pleasure. You may need to let go of the idea that intercourse is the only reason to have sex. This narrow idea of what sex is about may leave you or your partner feeling cheated. But during and after treatment for cancer, there may be times when intercourse is not possible, and you may need to explore other types of sexual intimacy. In fact, this can be an opportunity to learn new ways to give and receive sexual pleasure. You and your partner can help each other reach orgasm through mutual touching and stroking. At times, just cuddling can be pleasurable. You could also continue to enjoy self-stimulation. Do not deny yourself other ways of showing caring and feeling intimate because your normal routine has been disrupted.

Change Your Routine

Many couples have a favorite position for lovemaking or a routine for their sexual activity. If your body has changed with treatment for cancer, you may need to find new ways to be comfortable and to please each other. If your movement is restricted, or you are no longer comfortable in your usual lovemaking positions, experiment to find new positions. There is no right or wrong way. It is up to you and your partner to figure out what works for you both.

Sexual intercourse, and even physical pleasure, is not always at the top of everyone's agenda. Nonsexual touching—hugging, cuddling, or holding hands—is equally precious, and keeps couples feeling intimate with each other.

Address Upsetting Thoughts

Some thoughts are so upsetting that they can interfere with your desire for sex and cause you to change your behavior. For example, if you believe you are no longer attractive, you are unlikely to feel turned on, and you may discourage your partner's advances. In Chapter 8, we discussed common cognitive distortions, or thinking errors, and how to spot them. The power of upsetting thoughts can often be reduced by following these steps:

- Identify your feelings and the associated upsetting thoughts.
- Distinguish these from the actual situation that provoked them.
- Identify your cognitive distortions.
- Figure out another way of looking at the same situation that is more balanced but still believable to you.

When Not to Have Sex

Your health care provider will tell you when you can resume sexual activity after surgery. But whenever you are in doubt about whether sex might be harmful or hazardous, ask your health care team. The following are situations in which sexual activity may pose a risk:

❥ If there is bleeding in the genital area or urinary tract or if bleeding becomes heavier after sex, it's best to stop having intercourse until the cause has been identified and treated.

❥ If your immune system is suppressed or compromised, such as when the white blood cell count is low as a result of chemotherapy or radiation therapy, infection may be a threat. Ask your doctor if sexual contact would pose a risk of infection.

❥ If a man has any signs of sexually transmitted diseases such as a sore on the penis or whitish fluid (other than semen) at the tip of the penis, avoid sexual intercourse. To avoid the risk of an infection or a sexually transmitted disease, do not engage in unprotected sex if either you or your partner has other sex partners. This is more important than ever when one of you is undergoing treatment for cancer.

If you were critical of yourself before cancer, you may now have to face more ways in which you could potentially put yourself down. It may be hard to sort out the reality of the situation from your thoughts about it. You are more likely to make errors in your thinking when you are under stress, such as immediately after a cancer treatment.

Almost all of us put ourselves down as lovers now and then. The key is to become aware of your negative thoughts and see if there is another, believable way of looking at the same situation. Become more aware of what you tell yourself about your body and your sexual performance. You may be causing yourself anguish with thoughts like "A man with an ostomy is no good at all in bed." You can learn to reframe this as "A man who has an ostomy can make adjustments to have a good sexual experience."

When Is Sexual Counseling Helpful?

If you are experiencing a sexual problem as a result of treatment for cancer, you might find it helpful to discuss it with your doctor and other members of your health care team who can provide a referral to a specialist in sexual problems.

Such specialists are trained to provide therapy that focuses on improving a couple's sex life. Sex therapy is most useful if anger and conflict are not an issue, and the couple has a sound relationship and an affectionate bond. (If there is still tension and conflict in the relationship, standard couples' therapy may also be advised, since it is often impossible to separate physical responses from emotional ones.) Sex therapists help couples openly discuss and address their sexual issues, create closeness, and feel more comfortable exploring intimacy with each other through therapy sessions and at-home exercises.

Any sexual problem caused by anxiety can also respond to the counseling that a sex therapist provides. For women, problems caused by anxiety can include lack of desire, vaginal pain without a medical explanation, difficulty with arousal, and difficulty reaching an orgasm. For men, problems caused by anxiety can include loss of sexual desire, problems with erection that do not have a medical basis, trouble reaching orgasm, or premature ejaculation. Talk with your doctor to rule out a medical explanation for these problems.

If a medical condition is affecting a woman's sexual functioning, sex therapy may be useful to help improve her ability to respond to sexual touching. When a medical condition limits a man's sexual function, sex therapy can still be helpful, although the goals may be different. For example, instead of expecting a man to regain full erections, the therapist may help him and his partner learn to enjoy sexual caressing without erections. Sex therapists are also increasingly becoming involved in helping men and their partners decide whether to have medical or surgical treatments for erection problems.

Sex therapists may practice in a clinic or independently. Because most states have no laws regulating the title "sex therapist," a person with no formal training can call her or himself a sex therapist. A sex therapist should be a mental health professional (psychiatrist, licensed social worker, psychiatric nurse, licensed counselor, or psychologist) with special training in treating sexual problems.

Some Services Available

Different types of programs and specialists offer sexual counseling. The following is a partial list of programs and specialists that may be helpful (you can also ask your health care provider for a referral):

❥ **Sexual rehabilitation programs in cancer centers:** Cancer centers often have experts on staff who can evaluate and treat sexual problems. (Note that often these specialists see only those patients who are being treated for cancer at their hospital.) If you are being treated at a cancer center, check to see if such programs are offered there.

❥ **Sexual dysfunction clinics:** Many medical schools and private practice groups have comprehensive clinics to treat sexual problems. These clinics often provide both psychological and medical exams and treatments. The clinic staff may include psychologists, psychiatrists, social workers, urologists, gynecologists, and endocrinologists, among others. Some clinics require both sexual partners to participate in the evaluation, although you may be seen alone if you are not in a committed relationship. Some clinics offer a broader range of services than others.

❥ **Sex therapy:** Sex therapy is a brief type of psychotherapy (usually ten to twenty sessions) focused on solving a sexual problem. Sex therapists believe that a person learns lovemaking skills and that bad habits can be corrected by learning sexual techniques. In between meetings with the therapist, a couple (or sometimes just a man or woman treated alone) is given "homework" assignments. The homework consists of exercises to improve communication, develop more enjoyment of touching, and reduce the anxiety that can interfere with good sex.

A professional society, such as the American Association of Sex Educators, Counselors and Therapists (AASECT), can provide information about their members who practice in your area. You can also get a listing of sex therapists in your area by contacting your state's psychological association, a chapter office for the National Association of Social Workers, or state association for licensed Marriage and Family Therapists. There are also competent sex therapists who do not belong to any of these organizations (see the *Resource Guide* at the end of this book for contact information).

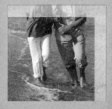

Chapter Eleven

Solutions
for Specific Problems

In Chapters 6 and 7, we discussed specific issues that can cause problems in a relationship. In this chapter, we look at problems such as infertility, and explore some possible solutions. We also look at extramarital affairs, divorce, domestic violence, and the abuse of alcohol or other drugs. We also offer ideas for dealing with the complications that can arise for people with cancer who are remarried or part of a dual-career or same-sex couple. Taking steps now to resolve these problems will help you and your family focus on confronting cancer.

Infertility

Difficulty conceiving children, whether temporary or permanent, can cause couples a great deal of emotional distress. Most couples usually assume that the choice to have children is theirs to make. When cancer or cancer treatment interferes with their ability to conceive, couples often experience grief and sadness. Even if the infertility is successfully treated, the couple may still find themselves dealing with the emotional impact of their inability to have children without medical assistance. However, by grieving the loss of having a family through a traditional way and then moving forward to create a family by other options, this loss can be eased in time.

Infertility resulting from cancer treatment often responds quite well to medical treatment. Additionally, there are several nonmedical options that can be explored, including adoption. Given the wide range of options, it is possible for almost any couple dealing with infertility to bring children into their lives. However, cancer survivors must face some difficult issues when deciding on whether to try to have children.

One important issue to consider is the potential impact of the cancer on life expectancy and on the ability to meet the challenges of parenthood. Uncertainty about whether cancer might return makes this issue a difficult one to address. Another issue that may play a major part in the decision to have children is family finances. Fighting cancer can drain a couple's financial resources. As a result, they may not be in a position to pay for the costs of either fertility treatments or adoption. Both of these options are expensive, and fertility treatment may not be covered by health insurance.

For these and other reasons, many couples who face cancer choose to remain childless. However, for younger couples who decide to have a family after cancer treatment, we will discuss a number of issues and available options.

Cancer Treatment and Fertility

Chemotherapy and radiation therapy can cause temporary or permanent infertility. Many factors can affect the likelihood that infertility will occur. Age is a factor for people who receive chemotherapy, and fertility often improves the longer the patient is off chemotherapy. Chemotherapy drugs that have been shown to affect fertility include busulfan, melphalan, cyclophosphamide, cisplatin, chlorambucil, nitrogen mustard, carmustine, lomustine, cytarabine, and procarbazine.

For patients receiving radiation therapy to the abdomen or pelvis, the amount of radiation directed to the testes or ovaries is a cause of infertility. For men, fertility may be preserved by the use of modern radiation therapy techniques and the use of lead shields to protect the testes. Women can have surgery to protect the ovaries by moving them out of the field of radiation.

Couples who are interested in having children should talk with their doctor *before* treatment to find out how it is likely to affect fertility. The doctor can then recommend a counselor or fertility specialist to discuss available options and help with the decision-making process. Some of these options are discussed below.

Banking Sperm, Eggs, and Embryos

Storing, or "banking" sperm, eggs, or embryos before going through a cancer treatment is one possible option for couples who would like to have children. Some of these options are more complicated and difficult than others.

Embryo banking is the most difficult of the three procedures. This requires a woman to take powerful hormone medications, and then embryos (eggs that have been fertilized by sperm) are surgically removed from her ovaries. This procedure is expensive, and the embryos may not survive long enough to be implanted after treatment.

Egg banking (with unfertilized eggs) is also difficult, especially since under normal conditions a woman only has one egg per cycle. This option requires the woman to delay cancer treatment and take hormone medications to stimulate egg production. Many eggs are needed because egg-freezing techniques are not perfect, and not all eggs will survive for future fertilization.

Sperm banking is much less difficult than the options available for women. It is typically offered to men who are having pelvic surgery, radiation therapy, or chemotherapy. With some cancers, however, sperm quality is affected even before treatment, so this option is not always successful. For instance, about 75 percent of men who have testicular cancer have reduced sperm counts and motility. Reduced semen quality can also be found in men who have had lymphoma or Hodgkin's disease.

Other Medical Options

If the nerves that control ejaculation are damaged in surgery, men may have a "dry orgasm." This is an orgasm that does not produce any semen. If this occurs, there are several things that may correct the problem. One procedure involves retrieving sperm cells directly from the testicle. Medications can be effective as well. For instance, ephedrine sulfate can sometimes stimulate the nerves around the prostate and the seminal vesicles so that semen will be released at orgasm. If a man has retrograde ejaculation in which semen shoots back into the bladder, sperm cells can sometimes be retrieved from the urine.

Research on the Prevention of Infertility during Cancer Treatment

Researchers are now exploring what can be done to protect a woman's ovaries from harm during cancer treatment, especially during chemotherapy and radiation therapy. Most of the trials have not been successful. There has been some success in giving women a long-acting hormone that induces a temporary menopause during treatment, but further research must be done to validate those results.

Researchers are also exploring taking a pool of sperm cells and preserving them prior to treatment. Most of the research needs to be repeated and validated by other studies before it becomes common practice in cancer treatment.

Radiation therapy or chemotherapy can often lower sperm count in men. However, it may still be possible to obtain enough healthy sperm after treatment and place them directly into a woman's uterus (intrauterine insemination) in the hopes that they will fertilize an egg. A newer technique, called intracytoplasmic sperm injection, can result in successful pregnancies even when only a few healthy sperm cells remain. With this technique, an egg is fertilized with a single sperm cell injected directly into it.

Third Party Reproduction

When someone outside the couple is used to provide healthy sperm or eggs, or to carry a child to term, this is called third party reproduction. These options may be attractive to couples who want to have the experience of childbirth or raise children who are biologically related to them. Before choosing one of these options, however, a couple must consider the ethical and moral issues that they raise. They also must consider practical issues such as how much contact a surrogate mother will have with the child or how much information the child should have regarding the history. With the many unique challenges and potential complications that third party reproduction poses, many couples are more comfortable using other approaches.

Adoption After Cancer

Adoption can be an attractive option for couples who would like to have children but would prefer not to go through fertility treatments. Unfortunately, the adoption process can be complicated by cancer; agencies may be concerned about the cancer's effect on life expectancy and parenting ability. Although the chances of a successful adoption increase several years after cancer treatment, some couples are still reluctant to inform adoption agencies about a cancer diagnosis. Private adoptions may be easier to arrange, but they can be very costly. International adoptions have become an increasingly popular choice over the last several years. They offer many of the same advantages as local private adoptions, but with less potential for legal disruption by the biological parents. If you are interested in adoption, try to get as much information as possible about your options before committing to a specific method.

PETER AND DENISE ALWAYS WANTED A BIG FAMILY but had not been able to get pregnant again after their daughter, Chloe, now fourteen years old, was born. After Peter was diagnosed with testicular cancer, he started a course of chemotherapy. Because of the treatment, his sperm count became too low to produce another pregnancy.

Their experience with cancer led Peter and Denise to feel that life was even more precious than before. However, they had been through enough medical intervention in the past year, and they didn't want to try fertility treatments. They both agreed that adoption was a great option. With Peter's positive prognosis, they were able to complete an international adoption within a year. Even though it meant some sleepless nights, they cherished the experience of raising an infant again, and Chloe was a doting big sister. Their new son, Miguel, was the light of their family's life.

Extramarital Affairs

Although issues related to fertility can be challenging, few things cause more damage to a relationship than extramarital affairs. An extramarital affair erodes the trust and commitment at the core of a long-term relationship. Repairing this damage can be a long and difficult process.

When a couple is dealing with infidelity in their relationship, they may find it helpful to see a therapist experienced in dealing with this issue. The therapist can help the person involved in an affair find an appropriate way to tell their partner about it. A therapist can also help the couple move beyond the affair and begin rebuilding their relationship.

In most cases, the first step towards healing the damage from an affair is to reveal the truth about it. Being honest about the affair provides one small step towards rebuilding the trust in the relationship. However, there are some situations when it might not be best to disclose an affair. Sharing the information may not be wise if it could lead to domestic violence. It also may not be helpful if there are already plans for divorce, as the information could be used against the person who revealed it. It may also be best not to disclose an affair that happened a long time ago. Often when such ancient history is revealed, it serves to ease the guilty feelings of the person who had the affair but causes unnecessary pain for the partner.

If you intend to tell your partner about an extramarital affair, there are several things to keep in mind. Although honesty is a good policy, there is no reason to tell your partner the vivid details about what went on in the affair. Giving a detailed description of the other person or discussing your feelings or your sexual relationship with the other person can result in your partner focusing on thoughts or images about the affair that are hard to erase. It will take time, usually at least a year, for your partner to move past some of the most painful effects of learning about the affair. During that time, your partner may experience intense feelings that will be difficult for both of you to face. Handling these feelings will require patience on your part and understanding that your partner will forgive you when he or she is able to. Trust takes a long time to rebuild, and it will probably be fragile for many years to come.

If you are the partner of a person who has had an affair, you must allow yourself time to heal. If you find that your reactions to the affair are interfering with your ability to enjoy life, it may be useful to see a therapist who can help you deal with your emotional pain. You should also take care of yourself, for example, by exercising and setting aside time to relax. Confiding in friends who understand what you are going through can also be comforting. Turning to family for support is more complicated because it could dramatically affect the future relationship between your spouse and your family. Even if you reach a point where you forgive your partner, your family may have a harder time accepting your partner again.

At some point, you will have to begin to trust your partner again. This can be difficult to do, as there is no sure way of assuring yourself of your spouse's fidelity. Even if it were possible to keep track of every waking moment of your partner's life, the time would be much better spent taking care of yourself.

At some point after the affair is revealed, it may be practical to see a couples therapist for help in tackling the problems that existed in the marriage when the affair began. Addressing these problems may take some time, as they will be complicated by the effects of the affair itself. (See Chapter 12 for information on how to choose a couples therapist.)

Doug and Mary have been married for eighteen years. They have three children and have weathered the usual ups and downs of married life. Four years ago, Doug lost his job. He became depressed and discouraged. It took him over a year to find employment.

DURING THIS TIME, MARY FOUND HERSELF looking outside her marriage for companionship, emotional intimacy, and a diversion from the dreariness of her life with Doug. She had several sexual encounters with a friend from work before she broke off the affair because she was so uncomfortable with her behavior. Mary felt it was important to have complete honesty in her relationship, so she told Doug about the affair.

Doug was devastated. His world as he knew it had been shattered. He felt betrayed and abandoned by Mary; however, he did not want to end his marriage or leave his children with only one parent. Doug and Mary saw a couples therapist for a year to try to heal some of the damage and distrust resulting from the affair.

Mary and Doug were making some progress towards healing their relationship, but it was slow. About two years after the affair, Mary was diagnosed breast cancer. Faced with the fact that Mary really needed his support, Doug was finally able to let go of his anger and hurt feelings about Mary's betrayal of his trust. At first it was difficult for him to shift his focus to being supportive, but Doug realized all the more how much he truly loved Mary. With this shift in attitude, he was able to understand why Mary indulged in the affair and began to forgive her for it.

Mary felt mixed feelings about receiving Doug's support throughout her illness and treatment. She had punished herself for years about the harm she caused to Doug and to their relationship, and she came to view Doug's lingering resentment as being what she deserved. But now that she had received what felt like true forgiveness from her husband, she was able to forgive herself. She was grateful to Doug for that and was all the more determined to be worthy of their renewed trust and intimacy in the future.

Divorce

A bout with a serious illness such as cancer can actually strengthen and enhance a relationship. However, it also puts a great deal of stress on both partners. Dealing with this stress can be particularly hard for couples with poor communication and coping skills. As a result, it can push a troubled marriage to the breaking point, leading to the decision to divorce.

Divorce requires each partner to make several major life changes. The process of going through these changes and adapting to them is complex and may take years. Although each person reacts to divorce differently, there are three major stages that most couples go through. Each of these stages involves specific challenges.

In the first stage, one or both partners begin to think about divorce. This stage often begins with one partner thinking about the possibility of a life separate from his or her spouse. This partner may then start investigating the possibility of getting a divorce and discussing this possibility with friends and family. The spouse wanting to change the marital situation may either avoid or confront his or her partner. This stage can involve a great deal of anxiety and even despair for both partners.

In the second stage of divorce, the couple addresses the practical aspects of becoming divorced. This stage begins when divorce is discussed as a real option. Once this point is reached, there may be a lot of turmoil in the relationship as feelings of fury, hopelessness, self-pity, or confusion are expressed. Sometimes couples are vindictive during this stage. Other times there may be a sense of relief at the possibility of a resolution to the marital problems.

Regardless of each partner's reaction, there are many decisions that the couple must make. If there are children, the couple must decide where they will live and how they will maintain contact with each parent. Another necessary decision is how the possessions will be divided. Often legal counsel or mediation is sought to help with such decisions. Mediation involves discussing issues that need to be resolved with the help of a neutral third party, often a professional mediator. The mediator helps the couple come to an agreement that each partner agrees is fair. If mediation is successful, it can prevent the need for a costly and often nasty court battle.

In the final stage of divorce, the basic decisions have been made, and each partner can begin to create a new life. The acceptance of the changes brought on by the divorce often comes with renewed energy and vitality. During this period, people tend to reach out to new friends and establish new activities. Sometimes as people explore new interests, they also get involved in new romantic relationships. Although this stage can be a period of growth, there is often lingering regret and pain about the losses from the divorce.

Rituals and special occasions can gain added significance after a divorce. Sometimes rituals can help in the adjustment process. For example, a person might burn a collection of old love letters to signify the end of one relationship and the beginning of a new life. Rituals can also be powerful reminders of the relationship that was lost. For example, holiday gatherings that include only part of the family can bring up intense memories and emotions—even in people who have adjusted well to a divorce. When facing occasions that were meaningful for the separated couple, it can help to prepare a coping strategy in advance. For example, a person might arrange to spend time with a supportive friend on the date of the couple's wedding anniversary.

Although friends and family can provide a great deal of support and helpful advice during the divorce process, professional help can be invaluable. Regardless of the stage of divorce, therapy can be helpful in several ways. A therapist can help a couple communicate their feelings in a safe environment. A therapist can also help couples stay focused on resolving the problems that they are facing, rather than blaming and battling each other. By showing and encouraging respect for each partner, a therapist can also help both people feel better about themselves. This can help build a sense of acceptance that allows them to move on with their lives (see Chapter 12 for information on how to choose a couples' therapist).

Therapists can also help people address complicated emotions related to the divorce. They can provide an objective perspective on what is going on in people's lives and help them find healthy ways to cope with all of the changes taking place. Many people find it helpful to see both individual and couples therapists while going through a divorce. If both partners are interested in individual therapy, it is generally recommended that they each see different therapists.

Domestic Violence

When you have been diagnosed with cancer, you need to treat the problem before it progresses to a more serious stage. The same principle applies to someone in an abusive relationship. The violence or abuse needs to be stopped as soon as possible to limit the damage it causes to the relationship and especially to protect the safety of the victim. The only way to guarantee that the abuse will end is for either the victim or the abuser to leave. Once this crucial step has been taken, it may be possible to correct the problem and begin to rebuild the relationship.

How to Help the Abuser

For abusers to change, they must first accept responsibility for their actions. They need to accept that nobody else causes them to be abusive. Although their partners may contribute to their anger, the decision to act with violence is the abuser's responsibility alone. If they are willing to accept responsibility for their actions and they are motivated, abusers can learn more appropriate ways to deal with anger and communicate their needs and feelings. Therapy is usually essential in helping abusers through this learning process.

Abusers often have many issues that therapy can help them to work through. The therapy generally focuses on teaching them alternative ways to manage anger. This includes developing a specific strategy for what to do if they start feeling out of control and angry enough to strike out at their partners. In addition to training in anger management, therapy can also help them deal with other problems that may contribute to their abusive behavior. These problems can include low self-esteem, jealousy, substance abuse, and problems with impulse control.

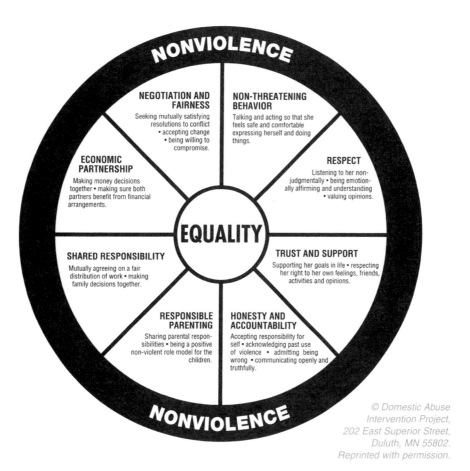

© Domestic Abuse Intervention Project, 202 East Superior Street, Duluth, MN 55802. Reprinted with permission.

Abusers can benefit from group therapy in addition to individual therapy. Once they have acknowledged responsibility for their actions, they may feel a strong sense of guilt and shame. By sharing these feelings with others who are going through a similar process, they may feel more able to take positive steps to improve the situation rather than blaming themselves for their past actions.

Couples therapy can also play a major role in healing the wounds in the relationship, balancing the power, and improving the communication between partners. Couples therapy is only recommended after the abuser has accepted responsibility and made substantial progress in handling anger appropriately.

While the cycle of violence revolves around power and control, as we described in Chapter 6, the *cycle of nonviolence* centers on a relationship based on equality.

Help for the Abused Partner

Safety is the first priority for people who have been abused. They *must* live apart from their abusers until the abusers have received the treatment necessary to resolve their behavior and have been nonviolent for a period of time. Before getting back together, both partners must agree that violence is completely unacceptable in the relationship. Even mild abuse can set the cycle of violence back in motion.

People who have been abused need a safety plan in effect, if and when they choose to live with their partner in the future. This plan should be detailed enough to allow them to act quickly and confidently if action is necessary. They need to develop a list of people who can help if there is an emergency and arrange for a place to go if abuse or threats occur. Keeping a second set of car keys available and a small amount of money ready is also a good idea. Finally, any firearms should be removed from the home.

People who are being abused must understand the serious risks of living with a batterer. They need to understand that they have no control over or responsibility for the abusive behavior. They also need to understand that batterers usually do not stop their abusive behavior without help from a professional and that abuse often gets worse over time. They may also need legal advice about reporting their partners' behavior. People who are abused must accept that their partners may not be willing to get the help they need to stop the cycle of abuse. If that is the case, they need to move on from the relationship and take care of themselves financially and emotionally.

Being the victim of abuse can have many effects on mental health, and it can seriously distort the way the world is viewed. Therapists can help people deal with these effects (see Chapter 12 for more information on therapy). The focus of therapy may be different depending on individual needs. People who are abused may need to work on making their own safety the highest priority, rather than trying to protect their partner's reputation. They may also need to learn new problem solving skills and more effective ways to communicate their needs to others. Group therapy can be particularly helpful in reducing the isolation that often comes from living in a home with domestic violence. By sharing their experiences and feelings with others who have lived through similar situations, victims of abuse can build connections with others and learn to recognize their strengths.

Alcoholism and Drug Abuse

In Chapter 6, we discussed how the abuse of alcohol and other drugs can affect relationships. Treatment options are available to help people or their partners with a dependence on alcohol or other drugs.

For the Alcoholic or Drug User

The first step in recovery for people dependent on substances is to admit they have a problem with alcohol or substance use. This usually happens because their friends and family confront them about the problem or because the results of their behavior are serious enough to force them to admit they have a problem.

Once a person realizes that he or she has a problem, the next step is to contact a therapist skilled in addiction treatment. The therapist can determine whether the addiction has progressed to the point where stopping the use of the alcohol or other drugs could cause withdrawal effects that need medical attention. If this is the case, the therapist may recommend hospitalization until the person's body adjusts to being substance free. Once this is done, long-term treatment can begin.

There are many programs that can help people who have substance abuse problems. The type of program to use is largely a matter of personal preference. People with more severe addictions tend to do better with programs that provide more structure, such as residential treatment programs. It is not at all unusual for people struggling with addictions to have periods of sobriety followed by relapses. Substance abuse programs often provide their clients with as many resources as possible to prevent relapse, and they also prepare them to cope with relapses when they occur without giving up hope of fighting the addiction.

For the Partner

Partners of people struggling with addiction often have many additional stressors to deal with. They may find that treatment and support groups can help them cope with these stressors more effectively. One support group that was specifically created for people who live with alcoholics is called Al-Anon. This group is based on many of the same principles as Alcoholics Anonymous, and it helps provide partners of alcoholics or substance users with a sense that they are not alone in facing the problems of living with an addict. The support provided by groups such as Al-Anon can be helpful whether the alcoholic or substance user is in recovery or not.

In addition to providing support, Al-Anon helps people identify how they can sometimes allow their partners to drink or use drugs without even being aware of it. Sober partners may help maintain addicted partners' lifestyles by assuming most of the household responsibilities and taking other steps to prevent them from suffering the consequences of their actions. When sober partners are able to recognize and change these patterns, they learn to live healthier lives and take better care of their own needs.

Although it is stressful to be the partner of an alcoholic or similarly addicted individual, it can also feel stressful when the partner has become sober. The presence of an addiction can affect the way each partner relates to the other, and they can both become accustomed to these ways of relating. When the addicted partner becomes sober, the relationship can change dramatically. For example, the addicted person may become more interested in participating in household decisions, requiring the nonaddicted person to adjust from being a caregiver to being an equal partner.

Couples in Recovery

Any change, good or bad, can cause stress in a relationship as each partner adjusts. When the addicted person is at an early stage in recovery, however, the focus needs to be on remaining sober. Once a person is stable in recovery, couples therapy can help take care of areas of the relationship that were neglected during the addiction and the changes that have taken place since the recovery began (see Chapter 12 for information on how to choose a couples therapist). Some of the issues that may need to be addressed at this point include:

❥ How to resolve conflict successfully

❥ How to talk about feelings

❥ How to make decisions and share power in the relationship

❥ How the couple can work to prevent relapse

❥ Who will do what tasks within the relationship

❥ How to let go of resentment over past experiences

❥ How to set specific goals for the relationship

In addition to adjusting to changes in responsibilities in the relationship, the nonaddicted partner may have various emotional reactions to the partner recovering from addiction. He or she may feel bitter about the events in the past that were associated with alcohol or drug use. The sober partner may also worry about "causing" the addicted partner to drink again, or have difficulty believing that the partner is truly in recovery. Rebuilding trust and adjusting to changes in the relationship takes time, and each partner can benefit from support during this difficult period.

KATHY HAS WORKED HARD AT RECOVERY from an addiction to alcohol and cocaine that she experienced while in her twenties. She is committed to her sobriety and is thankful that her husband, Nick, stuck with her through the hard times. She is now thirty-six years old, and she is currently undergoing treatment for acute leukemia. Although she has suffered with severe bone pain at various times throughout her induction chemotherapy, she has refused narcotic pain medications because she fears a relapse.

While Nick understands her concerns, he hates to see her suffer. To find a solution, Nick and the doctor consulted with a pain management specialist who also treats patients with addictions to create a treatment plan for Kathy. According to this plan, they will do what they can to relieve her pain, while also carefully watching for any signs of addiction. Once Kathy's chemotherapy is finished, she will be placed on a medication-tapering schedule that will gradually reduce her medicines without causing withdrawal symptoms. Kathy was reassured when she was told that patients usually do not develop dependence (either psychological or physical) to pain medications when they are used appropriately. With her husband and doctor's support, she is now being successfully treated for pain relief without risk of an addiction relapse.

Remarried Couples

As we mentioned in Chapter 7, almost half of all marriages involve people who have been married before. Families that result from remarriage are often called blended families. Blended families have more complicated relationships than traditional families. In blended families, couples need to act as a unified team to ensure the household functions well. This unity is especially significant when dealing with the added stress that comes with cancer.

In addition to unity, there are other characteristics that can help all of the members of a blended family be happy and comfortable and better cope with a crisis such as cancer. Two of the most important ones are flexibility and patience. Flexibility is critical for adjusting to all the changes that will occur in a blending of two families. It is likely that each family had their own ways of doing things, so everyone will need to make some adjustments in the new family situation. Patience is also valuable because the adjustment process can

Tips for Remarried Couples

Here are some specific actions that can ease the transitions of a blended family and help them cope with cancer:

❧ Try to resolve unsettled issues from your former relationships before remarrying.

❧ Set aside time as a couple to develop and nurture your relationship.

❧ Set aside time to spend alone with your children.

❧ When possible, negotiate the rules of the household with all family members.

❧ Decide before marriage how you will manage your financial matters.

❧ Allow the children and each other to grieve the losses of the original family.

❧ Take each change one step at a time—don't try to tackle all of the adjustments at once.

❧ Be as supportive as possible of the relationships between the children and their biological parents. Do not criticize or belittle your ex-spouse or your partner's ex-spouse in front of the children.

❧ Move gradually into a position of authority with your stepchildren—try to become friends first.

❧ When talking about cancer, let the children know (gently) that certain changes will need to be made in the family routine.

❧ Provide an open atmosphere for communication and sharing feelings and fears about how cancer is going to impact the family.

❧ Offer reassurance that things will get back to the way they used to be after treatment has been completed.

be slow and difficult. It will take time (probably years) for the new family to form its own rituals and identity, and the relationships formed may never be quite as close as those in a traditional family. Children in particular may have difficulty adapting to the new family and may often express these difficulties through behavior instead of words.

Dual-Career Couples

Dual-career couples often struggle to manage their commitments to work and family, as we discussed in Chapter 7. This can become especially difficult with the added strains and demands of cancer. When juggling the various commitments of work, family, and cancer treatment, it is easy for communication and the nurturing of a relationship to suffer. When fighting cancer, however, it becomes even more crucial to make sure you are available to support each other as a couple.

Dual-career couples often become self-sufficient and find ways to deal with their problems on their own. However, self-reliance may not be the most effective way to deal with cancer. The added demands on your time and energy that cancer treatment brings into your life will make asking for help essential to your well-being. The burdens of cancer shared with people who care about you may help to relieve some of your stress and allow you to focus on the more important aspects of taking care of yourself and your relationship during your treatment and recovery.

One area that can often be taken care of by other people is everyday household tasks. With income from two jobs, you may be in a position to hire household help to assist with these tasks. Or it may make sense to adjust your priorities and accept a slightly messier house, for example, in order to spend time together.

In a dual-career couple, there may be times that you need help when your partner is unavailable. It is useful to develop a reliable support network of people you can ask for help during these times. Having relatives and friends "on call" can reduce anxiety over what to do if an emergency should arise. It can also prevent feelings of resentment towards your partner who wasn't available at a needed time.

Often the biggest obstacle to getting help with the demands of cancer is a reluctance to ask for help. When people say, "Let me know what I can do," take them up on their offer and have a list of things to do ready. Your friends and family can offer a great deal of help with only minor inconvenience to themselves. For example, if you have children, there may be people who can easily bring them home from their activities. Or somebody who regularly goes grocery shopping may be able to pick up something extra for you. Small favors such as these can go a long way towards easing the burden of juggling work and cancer treatment, leaving you with some spare time to nurture yourself and your relationship.

In the Workplace

Many people are able to continue working while they or their partners are receiving treatment. Depending on the intensity of the treatment, there are several steps that you can take to prevent treatment and work from interfering with each other. It may be possible to schedule treatments late in the day or right before the weekend to minimize their effects on your work schedule. If treatment becomes demanding, you might consider adjusting your work schedule to ensure that you are able to take good care of yourself. You may find that it makes sense to move to a part-time schedule temporarily or begin doing more of your work from home.

If you need to take time off for treatments or to take your partner to treatments, discuss your situation with your employer (see page 24). Being open with your employer can have several benefits. What's more, there are federal acts that protect your rights while you or your partner are in treatment. Letting your employer know about your situation may make it easier to arrange flexible work schedules. It also allows you to prepare for absences to minimize any disruption to your work. One helpful activity is to make a log of your usual work schedule and duties so it's available when organizing any flextime, shifted duties, or time off. It may also be useful to include detailed responsibilities and instructions so that other people can manage your duties if necessary.

You can contact the American Cancer Society (800-ACS-2345; www.cancer.org) for more information on handling work-related issues, such as disclosing medical information to an employer, and the legal rights of people with cancer and their families.

Same-Sex Couples

As we discussed in Chapter 7, gay and lesbian couples face unique problems when dealing with cancer. There are several resources available that can help address these problems.

A number of factors may cause gay and lesbian couples to have a limited social support network. For example, they may have become disconnected from their family of origin due to their lifestyle. Or they may live in an area where homophobic attitudes are common. Joining a group or network that faces similar issues can help people feel less isolated and stigmatized. In many larger cities, special support programs led by therapists familiar with the specific needs of gay and lesbian couples are available. If such a support network does not exist in your area, the hospital social worker can offer information about other resources, such as gay or gay-friendly therapy or support groups, medical settings, clergy, or civil rights organizations. Taking advantage of available resources can provide a good source of support during a difficult time.

As with any couple, both partners in a gay or lesbian relationship may wish to participate fully in medical decisions. However, because gay and lesbian relationships do not have the same legal status as marriage, partners may not be given the same rights as a spouse to visit, participate in discussions with health care professionals, have access to medical records, or make decisions about health care. To prevent these problems, it is essential that legal documents detailing these rights be included in the patient's medical records. Partners should also keep their own copies of these documents. Legal counseling to make the necessary arrangements is often available through gay and lesbian community organizations.

WHEN LINDA WAS FIRST DIAGNOSED WITH CANCER, she felt isolated and alone. Although she had been with her partner Janelle for five years, Janelle often didn't know what to say or how to express her feelings. Linda also had many friends, but none of them had ever dealt with anything like cancer before. Her family was supportive, but lived far away. Janelle's family could not be relied upon for help because they did not know about her sexual orientation. Fortunately, Linda and Janelle live in a major metropolitan area that has a lesbian cancer initiative. This organization offers a weekly support group focusing on the needs and issues of African-American lesbians living with cancer. Through their involvement with this group, Linda and Janelle were better able to cope with the cancer diagnosis and treatment. Linda felt like this group was her lifeline as she was able to share her fears and doubts in a safe place with people she could trust.

The problems we discussed in this chapter can often pose serious challenges to relationships. In many cases, professional therapists can help in dealing with these problems. In the next chapter, we will give you specific advice on how to find a therapist who is right for you.

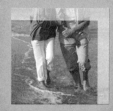

Chapter Twelve

Support
Services

A diagnosis of cancer brings a host of physical and psychological stresses. We have mentioned throughout this book that there may be times when you need to get professional support for problems that you are struggling with, especially if the problems are persistent and/or severe. Learning effective ways to cope with your emotional responses to these challenges can improve not only your well-being, but also that of your family and significant relationships.

In this chapter, we take a look at some of the resources that are available to support you and your family during a fight with cancer, including couples therapy, family therapy, support groups, and individual therapy. If you feel some hesitance about seeking therapy or support, remember that asking for help in dealing with cancer is not a sign of weakness, but a sign of strength. Finding resources for assistance is a way of taking control of your life and coping with what is happening to you.

Couples Therapy

Couples therapy (also called marriage counseling or marital therapy) focuses on relationship problems. It is different than individual therapy because the focus of treatment is on the couple's relationship rather than on a psychological

Support Programs and Services

There are many types of programs and support services available to help families during difficult times. Some programs, like support groups and group therapy, offer the opportunity to share what you are going through with others and develop skills or practical tools to cope with stress. There are also programs that offer financial and medical assistance. Here are some examples of available services:

❥ Individual, couples, family, and group therapy

❥ Support groups

❥ Home health nursing services

❥ Other social services such as financial assistance

❥ Nutrition services that provide meals or allow you to talk with a registered dietitian

❥ Rehabilitation services provided by physical and occupational therapists

❥ Spiritual support services from chaplains and other pastoral counselors

Making a decision about what is best for you depends on a number of things, such as what services are available from your hospital or community, the cost of services, and how you are coping with the illness. See the *Resource Guide* at the end of this book for more information about specific services.

problem within an individual. In couples therapy, partners identify problematic patterns in their relationship and then develop specific skills, as needed, to improve communication, resolve conflict, or enhance intimacy. We will discuss the various types of therapy that are available and then offer suggestions to help you decide if couples therapy is right for you and your partner.

When to Seek Therapy

When is it time to seek couples therapy? Many couples wait until their problems are dire and a separation is imminent before seeking help. It is better to catch the problems before they become serious and begin therapy before they have divided the couple. Here are some things to think about when deciding whether to seek couples therapy:

- **Do you need help communicating?** A couples therapist can often help you communicate more clearly, calmly, and objectively. This will make your discussions more fruitful and help you resolve disputes.

- **Do you find it difficult to support each other?** Couples therapy may be appropriate if you feel you need help getting to a point where you can act positively towards one another. Primary relationships should be ones in which at least some emotional needs are met. If this has stopped happening in your relationship, it's time to seek help.

- **Are there issues between you and your partner that are persistent and are affecting the quality of your relationship?** There may be a core argument (see Chapter 6) or particular issue that one or both of you cannot move past, such as whether to have children, or whether to move and where.

- **Is your sex life unsatisfying for either one of you?** Sexual intimacy is related to emotional closeness, and addressing problems in your physical relationship may help bring you and your partner close again (see Chapter 10).

- **Are you fighting a lot, without resolution? Is anger a part of your daily life? Do you no longer feel your home is a safe haven?** Problems can't get solved when anger is always in the air. A therapist can help you both diffuse the anger and identify some of the issues underlying the flare-ups between you.

- **Have you lost faith in your partner or faith in your unity as a couple?** Is one of you more deeply committed to the relationship than the other? If you feel that you can't trust one another, this can affect all areas of your shared life. Trust is the basis for intimacy. If one of you has started to back out of the relationship while the other remains committed, resentment will likely begin to build.

- **Do you feel that your partner doesn't listen to you or doesn't hear what you are really saying?** If you have tried repeatedly to express yourself and still don't feel understood, it may take a professional to help you figure out where the communication has broken down. There may be problems on the speaker's end, the listener's end, or both (see Chapter 8). A professional can offer specific skills that improve both sides of a couple's communication.

- **Do you feel you are drifting apart in your relationship?** We've talked about ways of becoming closer to one another emotionally (see Chapter 9). If those suggestions are not working for you, perhaps a therapist could help break down the barriers that are preventing more closeness.

- **Do you feel you can't be yourself in the relationship?** Do you feel powerless? You must be able to be yourself in the relationship (in a way that respects your partner's rights) to grow and thrive as a couple. If you feel your partner has all the power, it is a good idea to get help making the relationship equal.

- **Are you going through a major life crisis?** A preventive or supportive consultation with a couples therapist may be useful to help prevent stress from dividing you. Seeking therapy together may help enhance your communication and offer you an additional source of support so you can help one another cope in health ways while you are going through the crisis.

Before Taking the Plunge

Both partners should agree to try couples therapy. If one partner is resistant, it may be difficult to put the necessary effort into the process. That being said, therapy can still be useful even if one of you is reluctant at the beginning. The "right reason" for therapy can be simply that you are willing to try it out of respect for your partner. If the more eager partner presents some potentially positive reasons for seeking therapy, it may increase the likelihood of willing participation from the reluctant partner. Some examples of positive reasons are, "I would like to talk with you without getting angry," or "I would like to know how you feel about things." For couples therapy to be productive, any violence or abuse in the relationship must be addressed first (see Chapters 6 and 11).

Making progress in couples therapy takes a lot of effort from both partners. The process is likely going to require that each of you to give up your fantasies of your partner suddenly and magically changing his or her ways. You will both have to be willing to examine your own behavior and to compromise. Finally, remember that seeking help is not a sign of weakness or invasion of privacy, but a vote for your future together.

Specific Approaches Used by Couples Therapists

All forms of couples therapy involve learning how to improve communication so that couples can work together more effectively and have more fulfilling relationships. Couples therapy can teach partners to identify patterns of behavior that are harmful to the relationship and change those patterns. Each type of therapy described in this section offers a different way to achieve these goals.

In this section, we'll look at the most common types of couples therapy, with brief overviews of each theory and approach. Note that these are only summaries of complex therapies and the theories behind them. You may wish to ask your therapist for an in-depth explanation of his or her technique, either as part of a telephone inquiry or during the initial appointment. You may find that your therapist uses many different approaches or changes approaches during the course of therapy, depending on the goals you and your partner have.

No one method is right or wrong. However, you may feel more comfortable with some techniques than others and may wish to choose an approach that makes sense to you. The best indicator that the approach is right is if you feel that the quality of your relationship is improving as therapy proceeds; or, at the very least, that you are becoming more realistic in how you think about your problems.

Behavioral Therapy

Behavioral therapy is a type of couples therapy approach that focuses on teaching both partners new positive behaviors and helping them "unlearn" behaviors that are hurting the relationship. This type of therapy concentrates primarily on the present issues and does not usually address the history of the couple or of each partner. In essence, the approach aims to help both people reward each other more and punish each other less. Although this may sound simplistic, it can be quite effective when conducted by a skilled therapist.

Although you may think that it makes more sense to change how you and your partner feel about one another, it seems that as partners learn to behave differently, changes in their emotional responses to one another often follow naturally. In this type of therapy, you also learn ways to communicate more effectively or assertively. Home exercises are commonly assigned to the couple at each session. This homework often helps the couple practice a particular type of constructive behavior.

Behavior therapists may also use what are called cognitive (thought-related) techniques to work on reframing negative thought patterns and irrational ideas or *cognitive distortions* (see Chapter 8). These techniques can help partners think in a more balanced, realistic, or objective way about each other or their circumstances. Such mental strategies are used to cope with upsetting thoughts. For example, one person might think, "My partner is mad at me, so it's likely that she's going to leave." A cognitive approach would try to help this person look at the available evidence to see a more positive and reassuring perspective, such as, "When my partner has been mad at me in the past, she hasn't ever left me. She usually acts angry for a while, and later we can talk about it."

Psychodynamic Approaches

Psychodynamic approaches examine how early experiences may affect present relationships. Since our parents have both good and bad aspects of their personalities, we incorporate both into our personalities as we grow up. Psychodynamic approaches emphasize the importance of these internal images of our early experiences, and how we may come to view present relationships in ways that reflect these experiences. For example, we may be afraid of being abandoned by a partner if we felt neglected either physically or emotionally by a parent in childhood.

These approaches are similar to cognitive approaches in that they deal with the misinterpretations people make of their present situation as a result of their previous experiences. Cognitive approaches emphasize specific techniques to correct misinterpretations, whereas psychodynamic approaches emphasize the development of insight about the historical roots of present behavior and thinking. Psychodynamic therapies focus on developing a better understanding of our history, which allows us to view it in more impartial and objective ways. This can help us confront "ghosts from the past" and ultimately put them to rest.

Some therapists who use this approach may also suggest that one or both partners seek family therapy with their families of origin (parents and siblings) to address unresolved issues from the past. After such therapy, couples therapy can often be more productive.

MIKE KNOWS HE SHOULD BE MORE SYMPATHETIC to his wife Sara's inability to work during her radiation therapy, but he often finds himself sulking or losing patience when Sara experiences severe fatigue. Mike didn't realize until they spoke with the hospital social worker that he was afraid Sara was depressed because she was acting similarly to the way his mother had acted during her depressions while he was growing up. Seeing Sara immobile reminded Mike of how alone and hopeless he felt when his mother would lie in bed for hours instead of interacting with him and taking care of him. With the social worker's help, he was able to separate his experience with

Sara from what had happened with his mother, and once he realized that they were two different situations, he became less distracted by his fears of Sara withdrawing from him as his mother had. After that, he was able to be genuinely more tolerant and kind to Sara.

Family Systems Therapy

Family systems therapy also emphasizes the influence of our history with our families of origin. Just as psychodynamic approaches emphasize some form of "putting ghosts from the past to rest," the family systems approach emphasizes the importance of successfully separating from one's family of origin. This separation is called *differentiation* and is based on emotional, not geographical, separation. It involves seeing ourselves as independent and having more freedom to make choices rather than doing things that our families may have taught or expected from us. In this approach, one important question might be, "Am I repeating patterns of behavior that occurred throughout my family, from generation to generation?"

Another central concept of family systems therapy is that of triangles. You and your partner represent two corners of the triangle, while an outside party (such as one partner's family of origin) represents the third corner. Other outside influences that may become part of a triangle include things like extramarital affairs, problems with alcohol, or over-reliance on friends or family (see Chapter 11). The therapist in family systems therapy tries to "coach" the couple on separating the third party parts of their relationship and keeping appropriate boundaries with family members and with one another. The goal of this therapy is to be connected to each other while remaining an independent individual in the relationship.

ALICIA TALKS WITH HER BEST FRIEND about her marital problems with Keith because she feels like it is impossible to get anywhere with him. She didn't realize how much sharing this with a friend and not her husband harmed her marriage until her counselor pointed it out. She realized that because she was talking with her friend about the problems, she got some relief in talking about it, so she felt even less pressure to discuss it with Keith. Ultimately, she resolved she would share with friends only if she had made Keith aware of the issue first.

Communication Therapies

Communication therapies emphasize the present rather than the past. They focus on how families are organized and how current patterns of communication are affected. This involves looking at how the entire family is participating in and perpetuating a problem. The two basic methods of this therapy are called structural and strategic.

The structural method of therapy focuses more on how the structure of the family causes problems rather than on the problem itself. For example, a couple may avoid conflict between themselves by directing energy towards blaming their child for not doing homework. The problem really isn't about the homework; it's about the partners not facing their own dispute. This method of communications therapy attempts to change the way specific members of the family relate in order to bring about changes in the entire family.

The strategic method of therapy also involves examining the patterns of relationships, but it is more focused on the specific behavior patterns that need to be changed. This type of communications therapy is usually kept brief by setting clear goals to solve problems. It usually involves assigning tasks and homework. One technique sometimes used in this type of therapy is called *prescribing the symptom*. For example, a therapist instructs a couple who argue frequently to do so at least twice a day for a prearranged period of time. Both are encouraged to talk at the same time, interrupt each other, or do whatever else they tend to do that has been unproductive in the past. Under these circumstances, many couples reduce their arguments because they have conscious control over the "symptom" and discover that they no longer need to use arguing to communicate.

KIT AND SCOTT HAD A TENDENCY TO LASH OUT at each other when they were under stress. Scott just completed a long course of chemotherapy, and Kit was ready for life to return to normal. They were told by their therapist to give each other a good tongue-lashing for at least fifteen minutes a day. By the third day, they burst out laughing as they realized how ridiculous they sounded and felt. They feel their connection is much less hostile now.

Brief Therapy

Brief therapy typically involves ten sessions or less. Often therapists recommend brief therapy simply because insurance companies place limits on the number of sessions reimbursed. The objective of brief therapy is to identify one crucial problem or area to work on. The first session attempts to strengthen optimism and hope for both partners by emphasizing the couple's strengths rather than their weaknesses. With this type of therapy, the couple might focus on when they are *not* having a problem. Approaches similar to structural or strategic therapies may also be used. Since this therapy has a definite beginning, middle, and end, it might not be as intimidating to people who are otherwise reluctant to enter therapy.

Marriage or Relationship Enrichment

Marriage or relationship enrichment programs are those in which couples work in groups to learn specific skills and become more successful and harmonious companions. The key element of this process is a commitment to grow in the relationship, communicate more effectively, and resolve conflicts.

Like brief therapy, these programs tend to focus on the strengths of the relationship, and not just the problems. Skills in achieving the goals are practiced between partners and in cooperation with other couples. There are often marriage support group follow-ups in which couples can continue to meet and discuss issues with couples who have been through the program. Many marriage enrichment programs have a spiritual basis, although they may not be affiliated with a specific religious group.

How to Pay for Couples Therapy

Some insurance companies do not pay for couples therapy. That seems hard to understand, given that relationship satisfaction greatly affects your own and your partner's mental and physical health. If one or both of you have a diagnosis of depression or an anxiety disorder, therapy may be covered. However, couples therapy may still not be covered under these circumstances, so you should check with your insurance company.

Some mental health care providers offer couples a sliding scale fee, based on what they can afford to pay. In spite of this, there may be a limit to the number of sliding scale clients each therapist can afford to have.

How to Choose a Couples Therapist

Choosing a couples therapist can be as important as picking a competent oncologist. Here's how to start the process:

❧ First, choose a licensed professional who has both experience *and* training as a marital therapist. In general, a marital therapist should have a practice with more clients in couples therapy than in individual therapy. Trying to change individual behaviors versus helping couples live and love together are very different things. Don't expect one person to know how to do both. Specifically, you may want to ask the therapist about his or her track record—has he or she been successful with many couples—and ask the therapist to define success.

❧ Unless you have a specific agenda to the contrary, make sure your therapist is invested in trying to make your relationship work (rather than ending it). It makes sense for everyone to be working towards the same goal if this is the outcome you desire.

❧ You should both feel comfortable and respected with your therapist. If you feel either you or your partner is not getting respect, find another therapist. Also, neither you nor your partner should feel that your therapist is partial to one or the other side.

❧ There should be opportunities for you and your partner to voice your own values and goals for your relationship. If you feel that your thoughts and feelings are not valued or honored, try again with another therapist.

❧ Make sure that you and your therapist set achievable goals early on. You should not have to meet for a year before deciding that the approach is not helping. You should find the therapy helpful within the first few sessions.

❧ Most therapists understand that there should be a balance between addressing issues from your past and resolving current problems. If you feel you are spending too much time on the past and not the current problems, let your therapist know.

❧ The best way to get a good therapist is to be referred by another client. If you have friends that have had a good experience with a therapist, consider looking into treatment with that therapist.

❧ Last but not least, trust your gut. If you feel uncomfortable and can't put your finger on why, simply try someone else. It is your right as a client to halt treatment and change therapists at any time.

Even though couples therapy may be a major expense that you think you can't possibly afford, remember that you may end up facing more financial costs if your marriage dissolves. Couples therapy could turn out to be the best investment you ever made.

Support and Therapy Groups

Group support may be a good option for those who do not wish to become involved in couples therapy or for those who want something in addition to couples therapy. The purpose of group support is to help people in similar situations share their concerns with others and learn new ways to cope with problems. In a cancer support group, group members can expect to learn more about dealing with cancer and get new ideas from others.

One cancer survivor, Mary Ann, commented, "After treatment I found a support group to be an excellent resource to keep up-to-date on the latest treatments. We recently celebrated our tenth anniversary as a group this summer and invited our friends from the group to attend the celebration. There are seven of us that are breast cancer survivors of ten or more years."

Some groups are formal and focus on learning about cancer or dealing with feelings. Others are informal and social. Some groups are composed only of people with cancer or only caregivers, while others include spouses, family members, or friends. Support groups may also focus on specific types of cancer or even stages of cancer.

The length of time groups meet can range from a set number of sessions to an ongoing program. Some groups have open membership where people can drop-in without signing up ahead of time. This may be appropriate for you if you cannot make an ongoing commitment. Groups with closed memberships require preregistration and an agreement to attend a certain number of sessions. The benefit of this is that the same group members are present at each session, allowing for consistency and the opportunity for members to develop closer relationships with one another.

The three major types of groups are self-help support groups, therapy groups, and educational or coping skills groups. Let your needs help you decide what type of group is best for you. For example, if you feel isolated and alone with your illness, a support group may be just what you need. If you have problems with relationships or intimacy, a therapy group may be right for you. If you need information, such as how to explain your diagnosis at work or how to communicate with your doctor, an educational group will probably be most helpful. Or if you need to learn how to manage stress, a coping skills intervention group may be the best choice.

Self-Help Support Groups

Self-help support groups (also called peer support groups) are typically run by nonprofessionals who have been through similar experiences (they may be cancer survivors themselves, for example). Shared experiences and exchange of information are at the heart of this type of group. People who relate to your experience firsthand often have treatment-related tips that will be helpful to you. For example, they may offer a home remedy that was helpful with their nausea.

Studies have shown that support group participants have an improved quality of life, including better sleep and appetite. Not only is the peer network supportive, but it can also be fun and therapeutic. Laughing or complaining about the "weird" experiences one has as a cancer survivor is best done with others who have walked in your shoes.

Self-help support groups also give those recovering or recovered from cancer an opportunity to aid others who have cancer. With some training, many people with cancer find that helping others gives a boost to their own self-esteem. They may even become group counselors or facilitators.

Dolores shared the following reflections on her experiences, "I am a Reach to Recovery® volunteer. I share my own past experiences with cancer with someone who is facing breast cancer now. It can be very comforting to talk to a knowledgeable survivor who has already been through the experience. By sharing support, understanding, and up-to-date information, it helps calm the fears of newly diagnosed patients. It's a joy to hear the fear leave their voices."

Advantages to Being in a Support Group

❧ Support groups provide a feeling of connection to others during an experience that can feel isolating.

❧ They provide access to support during difficult times.

❧ You learn ideas from others about how they have made it through the experience you're facing.

❧ They help you feel less helpless because you are able to help others simply by showing up and sharing your experiences.

❧ They give you access to tips that only cancer survivors can provide.

❧ They allow you to voice strong emotions in a safe and supportive environment.

Choosing *when* to participate in a support group is important. Some find the period immediately following diagnosis a difficult time to join a support group. The stories that other patients discuss, after months or even years of treatment, can be overwhelming and upsetting. If you try a group and it doesn't feel right, you may want to try again at another time after you are further along in the treatment process. Or you may be able to find a more appropriate group for someone at your stage later on.

Therapy Groups

Therapy groups are different from the typical cancer support groups. These are professionally lead groups that offer therapy in a group setting. Therapy groups are often a good choice for people who have particular psychological issues related to their cancer experience. This might include those with a history of depression, anxiety, abuse, or relationship problems.

Therapy groups are lead by mental health professionals, such as social workers, psychologists, or other licensed counselors. The specific type of approach used by group therapists varies, and may include techniques such as interpersonal process, assertiveness training, or cognitive-behavioral approaches. Feel free to inquire with the group leader about what your participation would involve before deciding if a particular group is right for you.

Depending on the approach that the therapist/group leader is using, members may be asked to explore personal issues or practice particular skills as part of therapy. In many types of groups (especially those using interpersonal process techniques), participants are given feedback about themselves by other group members. Group participants are asked to set goals for the group that usually include changing something about the way they cope with certain situations.

Other Forms of Group Support

For those who cannot attend group meetings or appointments, counseling is also offered over the telephone by some organizations (see *Resource Guide*). Some people may find online support groups helpful because of the anonymity. It can be comforting to chat informally with other people facing similar situations. Chat rooms and message boards are often not the best source of cancer information, especially if they are not monitored by trained professionals or experts.

Regardless of the type of group you select, you should feel comfortable in the group and with the facilitator. If you have any fears or uncertainties about participating in a group, discuss them with the group's facilitator before joining, or as the group proceeds. And, of course, you are free to leave any group that makes you feel uncomfortable or does not seem to be helping you.

Individual Therapy

Sometimes feelings can be so intense that you don't feel comfortable discussing them in a group or with your partner present. You may feel so upset about your situation such that the idea of discussing it with others makes you feel worse. For people struggling with these kinds of feelings, or when marital conflict is intense or violent and it is not appropriate to proceed with couples therapy, individual therapy may be a better option. Once you have had some individual support and feel less anxious or overwhelmed about your situation, you will be in a much better position to benefit from a support group or couples therapy.

Individual therapy is an especially crucial first step if you are having problems with depression or anxiety. Depression can have a negative effect on relationships (see Chapter 5). A depressed mood may be due to cancer itself or unwanted adverse effects of cancer treatment; in some cases it may be a temporary, appropriate emotional reaction to stress. Or it may be a signal of a serious clinical depression that is more severe or prolonged than a typical reaction to stress and has no biological relationship to your cancer or treatment. It can be hard to tell the difference between these alternatives, so a thorough diagnosis by a mental health professional (preferably one knowledgeable about cancer and/or can consult with your physician) is essential.

It is especially important to consult a professional if you have a history of depression, your symptoms last longer than two weeks, or feelings of guilt, worthlessness, or hopelessness arise. If you have suicidal thoughts or are unable to eat or sleep for several days, call your doctor immediately. Prolonged depression that goes without treatment can deprive you of the quality of life that you are entitled to at any stage of illness, even at the end of life. Being depressed also complicates making reasoned, objective decisions about your life or treatment.

If you have problems with anxiety, it may also be helpful to consult a professional. Anxiety may be due to changes in the ability to function in family roles and responsibilities, loss of control over events in life, changes in body image, uncertainty about the future, or it may have a physical cause. Signs of an anxiety disorder include difficulty sleeping; physical problems such as sweaty palms, headaches, or upset stomach; recurrent panic attacks that lead you to change your lifestyle or lead to significant distress; avoidance of situations you would like to face; worry that makes you constantly tense or is difficult to control; or distressing thoughts that you cannot stop.

Like depression, anxiety disorders may be triggered or worsened by a prolonged or intensely stressful illness such as cancer. Anxiety disorders often go hand-in-hand with depression. Anxiety is an uncomfortable feeling. Fortunately, like depression, it can be treated in a variety of ways including medication, psychotherapy, a combination of both, or some other specialized treatment.

There is no reason to suffer with persistent emotional distress alone. The physical discomfort of cancer treatment is challenge enough without being disabled by depression or intense anxiety. Just as we encourage you to take the initiative in getting relief from your physical pain, we emphasize that treatment is available for prolonged or intense emotional pain, as well as distress in your relationship. Evaluation of your emotional care needs should be a part of your overall cancer treatment planning process. If you are coping well, you may still wish to seek out peer support as a way of preventing emotional problems or relationship problems from developing later. If you are overwhelmed, professional treatment—group, individual, or couples therapy—is available. We hope that the guidelines provided in this chapter help you decide which type of support or treatment may be best for you.

Couples' Corner

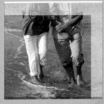

When two people fall in love and become committed to one another, they cannot anticipate the challenges or the joys that their relationship may face. Certainly cancer in one member of a couple puts tremendous strain on a relationship. This workbook contains exercises that are intended to help you cope as you struggle and grow together through cancer.

The exercises are written for all kinds of couples: those who have been together a long time, those who have recently started a relationship, those who are married or not married, whether straight or gay. We suggest you complete as many of the exercises as possible together, as a team, and that after you complete an exercise, you discuss it. Do them at your own pace and in your own way. You can add anything that seems right or skip any exercise that feels unhelpful or too difficult. Some of the exercises are designed to help you communicate better. Some of the exercises are designed to help with specific tasks (for example, dividing up chores in the family) or encourage you to discuss a difficult topic (for example, sexuality or death). All of the exercises are intended to help you discuss things that are meaningful or important to you as a couple.

Some of the exercises may bring up intense or upsetting feelings. We believe that strong feelings are normal and healthy during an illness (your own and your partner's). We encourage you to let the feelings happen. If the feelings get in the way of your coping, however, then we recommend that you talk to a mental health professional (see Chapter 12).

This workbook may be useful immediately after diagnosis, during treatment (you may even work on exercises in a doctor's waiting room or in the hospital), and after the treatment is completed.

Work together

Share together

Grow together

Learning to Listen

The goal of this exercise is to help you communicate more clearly and more respectfully with each other. Both partners take turns being the "speaker" and the "listener." As the speaker, you will learn to use "I" statements, as well as simplify and clarify your statements, so that your partner can hear the full message behind the words you are saying. And, as the listener, you will practice carefully attending to your partner's words and taking steps to make sure that you understand the message clearly.

This exercise takes practice and may seem awkward or simplistic at first. However, it is the most important exercise in the workbook and should be practiced first.

Take turns communicating a simple message. Each of you will have a role in this exercise. One partner will be the "speaker," and the other will be the "listener."

STEP ONE

Speaker: **Begin by communicating a very simple message.** Communicate simply and clearly. Only communicate one "chunk" of information, rather than two or three messages that are linked together. Begin your sentences with "I" rather than "You."

Speaker

EXAMPLE

"I'm feeling really sick today, and I would appreciate it if you would pick up take-out food for yourself and the kids."

STEP TWO

Listener: **Repeat what you heard your partner say,** rephrasing the message until you get it exactly right. After you repeat what you have heard, ask your partner if you fully understood. *This is not the time to respond to the message.* You will have a turn to respond to the message. Part of your job is to refrain from responding defensively, disagreeing, or arguing with your partner. Don't forget to ask your partner if you heard the message correctly.

EXAMPLE

"You said that you want me to get take-out food because you are too sick to cook. Is that right?" *Listener*

STEP THREE

Speaker: **Make sure your partner understood your message correctly and fully.** If not, *clarify the message.* Do not add any more information until your partner has fully understood the meaning of the first "chunk."

Speaker "Right, but it's not just that I don't feel like cooking, I don't even want to smell food cooking. I'm just too sick."

STEP FOUR

*Listener: **Again, repeat what you have heard,*** expanding on any part that is unclear, but not yet adding any information or responding in any way.

"So you don't want any cooking in the house. You want me to pick up some food for me and the kids." **Listener**

Speaker "Yes, that's right."

STEP FIVE

Continue to take turns speaking and clarifying until the message is delivered clearly and fully understood by the listener. Then trade places—switch roles. This is the point when the listener has a chance to respond to the message. It is now the speaker's turn to listen and not react. Take turns as speaker and listener, communicating simple messages until the technique feels natural.

Speaker "I know you want me to go out, but I'm too worn out. I'd prefer to make sandwiches or something that wouldn't smell up the house but wouldn't require me to go out again."

"You are tired and would prefer to stay in and make something easy. Is that right?" **Listener**

Speaker "Yes, but I am willing to make something that you won't have to smell, if that is helpful."

"You would prefer not to go out because you are really tired, but you are willing to prepare something that I won't have to smell. Thank you." **Listener**

Then and Now

A Picture of Our Early Love

Find a picture of the two of you, very early in your relationship. Post the picture here. Underneath the photograph, take turns writing down what you see in the other person that brought you together. (This exercise can be completed without a photograph; simply imagine yourselves together, early in the relationship.)

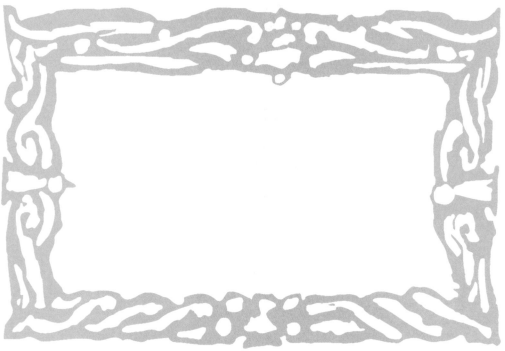

What attracted me to you then:

What attracted me to you then:

A Picture of Our Growth

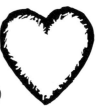

Post a recent picture of the two of you below. Take turns writing down what you see in the other person that keeps you together. (This exercise can be completed without a photograph.)

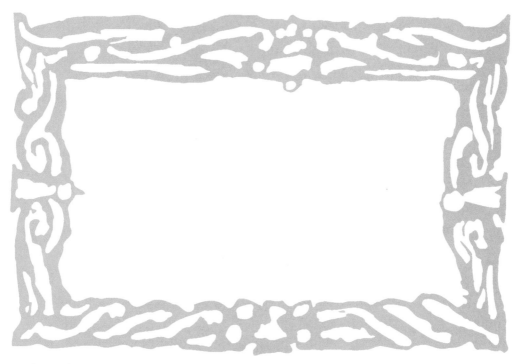

What I love most about you now:

_____

_____

_____

_____

What I love most about you now:

_____

_____

_____

_____

Circles of Feeling

It may be surprising to know that those with cancer and their partners feel similar feelings throughout the process of diagnosis and treatment. Your tendency may be to keep these feelings to yourself, but naming the feelings and talking about them can be very helpful, even if there is no simple way to make the feelings go away.

Identifying Our Feelings

STEP ONE
Choose a colored pencil or marker for each partner to work with. Each of you can use your own list of feelings from the following pages. Circle all of the feelings you have had since the first appearance of the cancer.

STEP TWO
Using a different colored marker or pencil, underline the feelings that are most difficult for you to cope with. For example, you may find that you are comfortable being angry but that anxiety is challenging for you to manage. On the other hand, you may be anxious much of the time, but when you become angry, you feel that you must resolve the problem quickly. Underline those feelings that are the most difficult.

Name:

Sad	Loved	Powerful	Enraged	Timid	Bewildered
Gloomy	Elated	Weak	Angry	Nervous	Confused
Despondent	Happy	Confident	Frustrated	Worried	Muddled
Blue	Cheerful	Insecure	Aggravated	Anxious	Concerned
Dissatisfied	Grateful	Competent	Mad	Apprehensive	Lost
Low	Satisfied	Adequate	Furious	Scared	Undecided
Displeased	Contented	Inadequate	Seething	Desperate	Vague
Off center	Devoted	Vulnerable	Irritated	Panicky	Torn/mixed
Desolate	Strong	Ineffective	Annoyed	Empty	Crazy
Anguished	Affectionate	Needy	Put out	Terrified	Silly
Cared for	Isolated	Inept	Violent	Disgusted	Laughable
Trusted	Committed	Needed	Desirable	Undesirable	Overwhelmed

Others:

Circles of Feeling

Name:

Sad	Loved	Powerful	Enraged	Timid	Bewildered
Gloomy	Elated	Weak	Angry	Nervous	Confused
Despondent	Happy	Confident	Frustrated	Worried	Muddled
Blue	Cheerful	Insecure	Aggravated	Anxious	Concerned
Dissatisfied	Grateful	Competent	Mad	Apprehensive	Lost
Low	Satisfied	Adequate	Furious	Scared	Undecided
Displeased	Contented	Inadequate	Seething	Desperate	Vague
Off center	Devoted	Vulnerable	Irritated	Panicky	Torn/mixed
Desolate	Strong	Ineffective	Annoyed	Empty	Crazy
Anguished	Affectionate	Needy	Put out	Terrified	Silly
Cared for	Isolated	Inept	Violent	Disgusted	Laughable
Trusted	Committed	Needed	Desirable	Undesirable	Overwhelmed

Others:

How We Can Cope with Our Most Difficult Feelings

This part of the exercise is designed to help partners understand the wants and needs of the other when their feelings are strong or difficult to handle. For example, some people want to talk when they are angry, whereas others want some time to cool off. Some people want advice or help problem solving, but many people do not want advice—even if they want to talk about their anger. Many would prefer simply to be listened to, as demonstrated in the *Learning to Listen* exercise. People have different needs when they are sad as well. Some people want to be held or comforted, whereas others prefer a few minutes alone to work out their feelings. Some people like to write or draw pictures when they are sad, before they can talk about their feelings.

    Clarifying your own needs and practicing communicating them to your partner is the goal of this exercise. Designate an area for each of you. Write down two difficult feelings from your feelings list. After each word, write down at least one thing that you would like from your partner when you feel that way. Share the feelings and your own preferences with your partner. Next time you have that feeling, let your partner know what you are feeling, and remind him or her about what would be helpful.

Partner's Name:

Feeling	Way of Coping
Feeling	Way of Coping
Feeling	Way of Coping

Partner's Name:

Feeling	Way of Coping
Feeling	Way of Coping
Feeling	Way of Coping

Still Kids Together

When people are ill, they often think about their lives in new ways and with new perspective. Many people ponder some of their childhood memories—both happy and unhappy. It can bring you closer together when you share these memories and their meaning with one another. Obviously we cannot relive our childhoods. However, it is possible to identify the most meaningful elements of our childhoods and to try to recreate those meanings in our current lives. The first goal of this exercise is to share a few happy or meaningful childhood memories with your life partner. Next, you will identify the elements of these memories that are most important, and think about how you can recreate some of these early feelings in your current relationship.

STEP ONE

Individually, take a separate sheet of paper and record two or three of your most significant childhood memories. In this exercise, choose memories that are positively meaningful to you. Examples may include favorite family events, rituals, or holidays, or time with a favorite friend or relative.

STEP TWO

Next to each memory, record the most important element of the event. Answer the question, "What was it about this event that was so meaningful to me?" Also record the main feeling that was associated with the memory. Use the feeling list from the earlier exercise to help describe your feelings.

STEP THREE

Take turns sharing memories with your partner. Tell the story of the memory fully. Share it in detail and describe the feelings and the meaning of the memory. Your partner may have a similar memory to share.

EXAMPLE

JACK REPORTED A FAVORITE MEMORY of spending time with his siblings. His siblings are now spread across the country and have not been together for several years. He described this memory, "My whole family was camping in Virginia. We had this huge old tent. My parents were taking a walk and the four of us decided to have a picnic INSIDE the tent to surprise my parents. We put the picnic table inside the tent with a cloth over it, and my sisters got all excited, running around making drinks and sandwiches. The meal was nothing, but we were just together, excited and spontaneous. No one tried to make it perfect, that's what mattered to me. And my parents didn't really even get it, but we didn't care. I felt young and free and part of a family. I miss that."

STEP FOUR

This is the creative part of the exercise. Work together. Your goal is to find some simple way to recreate the essence of your experience in your current life together. You will never recreate your childhood, of course, and that is not expected. So try not to be skeptical. The goal is to allow yourself a few moments of freedom, to honor a memorable time in your life, and to share that experience with your life partner.

EXAMPLE

JACK WAS IN THE MIDDLE OF HIS TREATMENTS for lymphoma. He had completed several rounds of chemotherapy and had difficulty eating. His energy was typically low except in the late afternoons, when he joined his wife and two children for dinner. After completing this exercise, he and his wife decided to have a picnic for their next meal with their kids. His wife, Sarah, with the help of their fourteen-year-old son, brought the lounge chairs into the living room, and the whole family ate at the coffee table. Jack had yogurt, but the rest of the family ate sandwiches. After dinner, everyone drank hot chocolate, and Jack and Sarah shared two of their favorite memories with their children. Their goal was not to "try to make it perfect, just to be spontaneous, free, and part of a family."

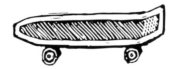

Runners and Chasers

As discussed in Chapter 3, couples can sometimes "polarize," or take on opposite roles, in their communication styles, particularly when they are in conflict or under stress. In polarized conversations, one member of a couple will become the pursuer or "chaser," while the other will withdraw or become the "runner." The chaser will go after the runner, trying to discuss difficult topics, while the runner avoids conflict at all costs. Chasers may feel that their partners are avoiding them personally and feel rejected. At the same time, runners often feel picked on or criticized by their partners' persistent efforts to talk about things.

Working with Your Communication Style

Your communication style may not be a problem during regular times. However, coping with cancer requires a tremendous amount of problem solving, which can tax the resources of even the healthiest couple. While dealing with illness, couples may become rigid in their conflict styles and fall into painful and undesirable patterns of communicating.

As a couple, use the Communication Style Checklist on the next page to help each of you to indentify your conflict style. The runner and chaser checklists are followed by worksheets and exercises (pages 226–229) to help you communicate more effectively.

Put your initials by each statement that is true (or somewhat true) of your behavior in conflict.

COMMUNICATION STYLE CHECKLIST

Chaser Checklist

☐ When I am upset, I want to discuss it immediately, or as soon as possible.

☐ I cannot go to sleep in the middle of an argument. I prefer to resolve things first.

☐ When I have a problem to solve, I like to solve it as a team.

☐ When we argue, I want to keep talking until we resolve things and feel close again.

☐ When my partner is angry with me, I find myself wanting to move closer in order to "make peace."

Runner Checklist

☐ When I get angry or hurt, I need some time by myself to cool off.

☐ When my partner and I argue, I often want to "sleep on it" and work it out later.

☐ I believe that things often work out better if we just leave them alone.

☐ I prefer to solve problems by myself and discuss them later.

☐ When my partner is angry with me, I usually want to be left alone.

If you checked three or more items on either the runner or the chaser checklist, this is probably the typical conflict style you use with your partner.

The following worksheets may be helpful to you during your next conflict. Take a few minutes now to review the worksheet that corresponds to your conflict style. Next time you find yourself in this pattern of running and chasing with your partner, pull out the worksheet and follow the steps.

Runners and Chasers

Worksheet for the Chaser

STEP ONE

When you and your partner have had a dispute, tell your partner that you are upset and that you plan to do some writing about your conflict. Ask your partner if he or she would be willing to discuss the argument with you again at a specific time, after you have cooled off and collected your thoughts.

STEP TWO

Write down exactly what you are angry about right now. What did your partner do specifically that upset you? Don't hold back. This is your private anger page. You will not share this page with your partner. You may wish to use a separate page for your journaling or to begin writing in a bound journal to keep for future conflict resolution.

STEP THREE

Ask yourself these questions: "What are the fears behind my rage?" "What am I really afraid of?"

STEP FOUR

Ask yourself these questions: "What hurt my feelings?" "What were the hurts behind the anger?" "How did I feel slighted or unloved in our interaction?"

STEP FIVE

Share your fears and hurts with your partner. Use the *Learning to Listen* technique to talk about your feelings. Take turns and ask your partner to reflect on what you said.

Runners and Chasers

Worksheet for the Runner

STEP ONE

When the conflict becomes too intense and you need some time off, ask for a "time out" and set an appointment to talk later. Because you are the runner, it is your responsibility to make an appointment to talk again. If you don't, your partner is likely to keep chasing you, and you won't have a chance to cool off.

One common mistake that runners make is that they ask for a break in a way that blames the other partner. (For example, "Leave me alone, you're driving me crazy.") If you really want a break, you will have to ask for it directly. You also need to set a time to resume the discussion and approach your partner at that time. Try this request, "I need a few minutes to cool off so that I can communicate with you more effectively. Let's talk again in __ minutes."

STEP TWO

Take half of the "time off" to cool down. Take a walk, rest, or work on a project that puts you in a good mood. Then return to the exercise and complete Step Three.

STEP THREE

Write down exactly what made you angry in the conflict with your partner.

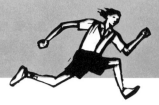

STEP FOUR

Ask yourself these questions, "What are the fears behind my rage?" "What am I really afraid of?"

_____

_____

_____

_____

_____

STEP FIVE

Ask yourself these questions, "What hurt my feelings?" "What were the hurts behind the anger?" "How did I feel slighted or unloved in our interaction?"

_____

_____

_____

_____

_____

STEP SIX

Share your fears and hurts with your partner. Use the _Learning to Listen_ technique to talk about your feelings. Take turns and ask your partner to reflect on what you said.

Our Greatest Fears

This exercise can be completed together or separately. The goal of this exercise is to identify your greatest fears about cancer and share them with each other. The goal is not to hide or minimize the fears, but to claim them as your own and begin to communicate them to one another.

STEP ONE
The following page has six shapes. Each partner should choose three. Inside the shape, record one of your greatest fears related to cancer.

EXAMPLE

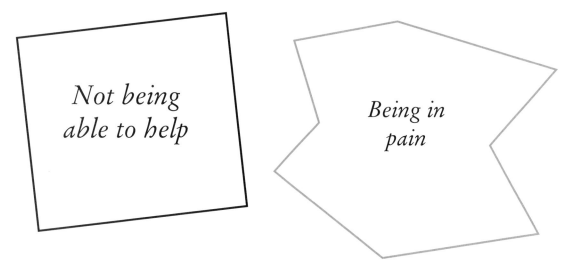

Not being able to help

Being in pain

STEP TWO
Choose one of these fears to discuss with your partner using the communication exercise *Learning to Listen*. Remember that as you listen to each other's fears, it is not your job to make the other feel better, but simply to listen and try to understand. You may find that your fears are similar. Later exercises will help you find ways to manage your fears.

Let's Make a Deal

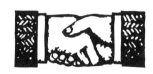

Use this technique when you are in need of help but feel too ashamed or afraid to ask. During the experience with cancer, both the partner who is ill and the caregiver often feel burned out and exhausted. It is difficult to ask for help when you know your partner is tired too. This technique may make it easier to ask.

Keep in mind that *Let's Make a Deal* is a game. The goal of this exercise is to make a request in a playful and light-hearted way. The deal does not need to be sensible or even fair. By asking your partner to make you a deal, you are acknowledging that you are asking for a favor, and you at least *wish* that you could return the favor.

EXAMPLES

"I'll make you a deal. If you do the dishes the rest of this week, I won't complain about anything for the first twenty minutes when you come home from work each night."

"I'll make you a deal. If you get the kids ready for school in the mornings, I'll make the beds."

"Let's make a deal. If you rub my shoulders, I'll tell you the whole story of our honeymoon, including all the details."

"Let's make a deal. I'll take over all of the cleaning of the house, if you'll try not to take it out on me that the treatments are getting more difficult. I don't mind hearing how hard it is, how sick you feel, but just try not to snap at me quite so much."

Can Cancer Be Funny?

Many cancer survivors report funny stories—ridiculous things that happened to them during their illness and/or treatment. Often these incidents have meaning for the cancer survivor and family members. Most days, though, cancer is not funny. But as we discussed in Chapter 4, finding humor in difficult circumstances can be the best medicine for your relationship. Save this page—just in case you have an incident that you want to record and remember.

EXAMPLE

SARAH AND HER PARTNER MARTHA WENT TO THE GROCERY STORE immediately after her fourth chemotherapy treatment for lymphoma. She became nauseous in the store and had to sit on a bench with her head between her legs, while Martha went to get the car. Martha was seventy-five years old and suffering from arthritis, and she was afraid she would be unable to help Sarah to the car. So Martha, being a problem-solving type, rounded up a motorized cart in the grocery store and loaded Sarah into it. Sarah immediately put her bald head between her legs so she wouldn't faint, and Martha drove her to the car. Sarah tells this story giggling and crying because she remembers all of the people in the grocery store gathering around trying to offer support to the "old lady and the bald woman in the motorized grocery cart." This was the day that Sarah remembers realizing that "no matter what happens, people will help."

If you have funny or meaningful incidents that you want to remember, record them here. Read the story to your partner, and encourage him or her to record a story as well. Many people with cancer and their partners keep journals of their experiences. This may be a good time to begin yours. After you record your funny story, describe what the incident meant to you as a couple.

Today Cancer was Funny

Our Support

For many people with cancer, one of the biggest challenges is asking for help. People with cancer may need transportation to and from the doctor, assistance during treatments, help with childcare, meal preparation, physical assistance in the home, as well as other needs. Often the caregiver must arrange the help.

Some people with cancer and many caregivers resist asking for help because of messages they received from their past, such as "Be independent," "Keep your chin up," or "Don't talk about your problems outside the family." Some of these messages are part of our families or culture. It may be helpful to discuss these old beliefs or messages with your partner (see Chapter 3). Yet cancer forces us to put aside some of these early messages and ask for help anyway. Interestingly, people who are asked to assist a neighbor or friend during a time of illness often report that they feel valued and appreciated. People often find meaning and pleasure in being able to help others.

In this exercise, work together to develop a list of potential helpers, and discuss what roles you might ask each person to fill. We suggest dividing helpers into three levels of care:
1. *Neighborly support* (bringing meals, picking up mail, filling prescriptions, and so on)
2. *Friendly support* (transportation, help with children, being available to call in case of emergency, administering medications, and so on)
3. *Close support* (assistance during treatments and treatment-related illness, physical assistance in the home, updating family and friends)

List every single person who comes to mind using a chart similar to the one below. Do not cross anyone off the list unless being with him or her would be exhausting. Even an acquaintance or friendly neighbor may be able to provide some level of support.

Next, identify what "level of care" you feel comfortable requesting from this individual. Then, identify tasks that you might ask them to help with. Finally, identify which of you will ask for this help.

OUR SUPPORT	LEVEL OF CARE	TASKS	WHO WILL ASK

Just from You

As discussed in the previous exercise, asking for help can be difficult for people with cancer and their caregivers. There may be some special responsibilities (talking with family members, for example) that you would prefer your partner to help with, rather than a friend or neighbor. It can be practical to identify these tasks, so that your partner can prioritize his or her time and energy.

What Do I Need Just From You?

This part of the exercise is for the partner with cancer to complete. List below any things that you would like your partner to take care of, instead of asking a friend or neighbor. Try to limit the list to one or two tasks, and be realistic of your partner's time constraints. It may not be reasonable, for example, to ask your partner to accompany you to every treatment. But it might be important to have him or her at the first appointment.

What Can I Do?

This part of the exercise is for the caregiver to complete. Think through which of the above tasks you can do with relative ease. If there are requests on the list that will be difficult for you, talk with your partner about why that behavior would be hard for you. Next, work together to consider other options.

EXAMPLE

PATRICK, WHO WAS RECENTLY DIAGNOSED WITH A MALIGNANT BRAIN TUMOR, asked his wife Mary if she would be willing to tell his elderly mother about his illness. Mary wanted desperately to help Patrick in any way possible; however, she did not feel that she could talk with Patrick's mother alone because she was afraid that she would break down and be unable to explain the illness to her adequately. When they discussed Mary's fears, the couple decided that Mary would tell Patrick's sister, and that the two of them (Patrick and his sister) would inform their mother together. This worked well, because Patrick's mother had someone to lean on when she heard the news.

Simple Pleasures

As a couple confronting cancer, your romance may be at its peak, or it may be suffering due to the tremendous demands on both of you. This exercise is designed to reintroduce small gestures of romance into your relationship.

STEP ONE
On separate sheets of paper, make a list of small things your partner does regularly that please you and make you feel loved or "courted." List everything you can think of. Stick to the small things, such as holding your hand in the car or at the doctor's office, kissing you at the end of the day, pouring your coffee in the morning.

STEP TWO
Add to the list any behaviors from earlier in your relationship that brought you pleasure (leaving a note or card, calling during the day to check in).

STEP THREE
Add three small things you wish your partner would do more often or just once or twice. These should be from your imagination (bring home a rose, rub your feet, talk to family members when they call, dance with you in the living room, read a favorite story or poem to you).

STEP FOUR
Rank the behaviors by how much pleasure they bring you. Rank the most pleasurable behavior as number one.

STEP FIVE
Exchange lists. Without discussing it, try to do one thing from your partner's list each day. If you or your partner is too tired or ill to do anything on the list, tell your partner what you would do if you weren't tired. For example, say to your partner, "I'm imagining rubbing your feet right now. I would love to do that for you."

Must We Talk about Death?

Should you be talking about the possibility of death? Do you need to begin talking about it now?

Although many cancers are treatable, people with cancer and their partners almost always think about death in a way that is closer to home than ever before. Regardless of whether your cancer is life threatening, it may be valuable to talk about the possibility of death—both for practical reasons (writing a will, creating a living will, or making medical decisions for example) and for emotional reasons (sharing your thoughts and fears with your partner and avoiding isolation about an upsetting topic).

Use the following list of questions to begin discussing death with your partner. If this topic is too painful or not relevant, skip this exercise. But if it is constantly in the back of your mind, try to talk about a few of the questions now. You can return to the exercise at a later time if you find yourself thinking about death or dying.

Take one question at a time. Ask your partner the question and listen to the response using the *Learning to Listen* technique in the first exercise. Then switch roles and respond to the question yourself before moving on to the next question.

1.   *Do we need to discuss the possibility of death? Is it likely that you will die?*
2.   *If so, do we need to talk about it now? If not now, when?*
3.   *What is the most difficult thing about discussing death?*
4.   *What can I do to make it easier for us to talk about it?*
5.   *What questions do we need to ask our health care providers about death?*
6.   *If death is a strong possibility, whom do we need to inform? Should we begin a list of whom to inform now?*
7.   *How do you want to inform family and friends about your illness?*
8.   *Is it time to begin talking about hospice care or other long-term care?*
9.   *How and where do you want to die?*
10. *Do we need to have our wills/living wills, power of attorney, and other paperwork written or updated? How should we start this process?*
11. *What do you believe happens to a person after death?*
12. *What do you want to happen at your funeral/memorial service?*
13. *Do you want to be cremated or buried? Should we make arrangements now?*
14. *How do you want to say good-bye to me? What is most important for us to do together before you die?*

Questions of Spirit

Cancer challenges every relationship. It can also challenge one's relationship with God or a higher power. Some people with cancer report a renewed sense of peace, or a broadened, deeper sense of spirituality. Many others report anger and confusion about their spiritual beliefs.

As a couple, you may share religious or spiritual beliefs, or your beliefs may be very different. This is a good time to think about your beliefs and to share your spiritual journey with your partner. Complete each of the following sentences individually, and then share your responses with your partner.

I believe in _____

I do not believe _____

When I think about my spirituality I feel _____

The place where I feel most at peace is _____

I feel closer to God or a higher power when I _____

As a child I believed _____

My family's beliefs were _____

I feel most spiritual when _____

Since cancer, my relationship with God or a higher power _____

My spiritual goal is _____

I believe that when I die _____

The best way that my partner can support my spirituality is _____

Three to One

Research on couples' communication suggests that most people can only tolerate hearing one criticism at a time. Furthermore, people tend to respond most positively to constructive criticism when it is presented in the context of positive feedback. Some couples' therapists suggest a ratio of three positive comments about your partner for every one criticism or request for change.

Three Successes and One Request

On separate sheets of paper, write down three ways you believe that both of you, as a couple, are dealing with cancer well. Next, write down one way in which you wish your partner would deal with you differently. Be sure to make it a request for your partner to "do something" rather than to "stop doing something." For example, rather than asking your partner to "stop yelling at me when you are angry at the doctors," ask your partner to "speak to me in a normal tone of voice, even when you are angry with the doctors." As another example, rather than asking your partner to "stop leaving dirty clothes on the floor," ask your partner to "put your dirty clothes in the hamper please."

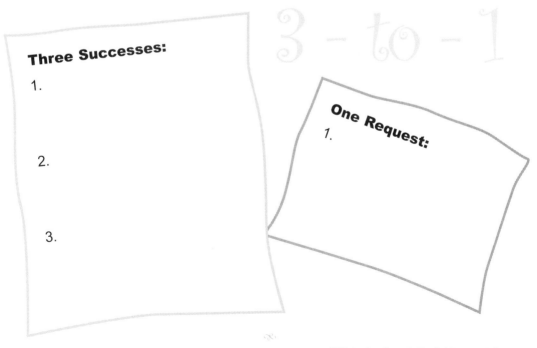

Three Successes:

1.

2.

3.

One Request:

1.

Getting the Most from Sex

Inevitably, cancer affects a couples' sex life. It forces many couples to discuss sex, when they have tended in the past to "just do it." Talking openly about sex and sexuality can be awkward, but it can also be highly rewarding and even exciting. And it can make it possible to adapt your sexual behavior with one another so that you remain sexually alive and connected, even if your sex life has changed drastically, as we discussed in Chapter 10.

Sexual satisfaction comes from being able to talk openly and honestly about what you want and how you want it. With cancer, this may include talking about what you can no longer tolerate. For example, it may mean asking for gentle physical affection rather than intercourse or oral sex. The purpose of the following exercises is to help you, as a couple, discuss the changes and challenges that cancer has brought to your sexual relationship and what you can do to improve it.

Talking about Changes in Our Sexual Relationship

On separate sheets of paper, write down three ways that cancer has affected your sexual relationship. Next to each change, write down your feelings about the change. Refer to the feeling list on page 219 for words to describe your feelings.

Discuss these changes and your feelings about these changes with your partner. If there is a loss of sexual desire or ability to be sexual as before because of physical changes or fatigue, discuss what this loss means to you.

CHANGES IN OUR SEXUAL RELATIONSHIP
1. Change:
Feelings:
2. Change:
Feelings:
3. Change:
Feelings:

CHANGES IN OUR SEXUAL RELATIONSHIP
1. Change:
Feelings:
2. Change:
Feelings:
3. Change:
Feelings:

Requests for Intimacy and Affection

Write down three things you would like to ask of your partner. Make these requests for your partner to "do something," rather than to "stop doing something." For example, you might ask your partner to "touch me gently and slowly around my radiation areas," rather than "don't touch me so hard."

Some requests may need to be made in the negative, particularly those regarding medical instructions or orders from a doctor. In those cases, be clear and direct about what you need and want. For example, you may need to abstain from intercourse during and after some forms of treatment. Avoid confusion or misunderstandings by informing your partner of these precise requirements. Refer to Chapter 10 for specific suggestions and guidelines for talking with your doctor or other health care professional about sexuality and cancer.

Personal requests for behaviors that are traditionally sexual (related to sexual intercourse or oral sex) or related to other forms of affection (holding hands, kissing, massage, and so on) may also be requested on your list.

REQUESTS FOR INTIMACY AND AFFECTION	REQUESTS FOR INTIMACY AND AFFECTION
1.	1.
2.	2.
3.	3.

Exchange lists with your partner. Discuss which of the things on your partner's list you can do with relative comfort and which of the requests seem too intimidating or difficult. Modify the lists to include three important changes that you and your partner would like to bring to your sexual relationship.

241

A Collage of Pictures and Words

MATERIALS: Poster board, glue sticks, scissors, colored markers, magazines, pictures, and so on.

This is a good exercise to do together. If you wish, the caregiver can provide the materials and labor, while the partner with cancer can work at his or her own pace.

Imagine the poster board in three sections—past, present, and future (see below). From magazines or other sources, cut out pictures, words and symbols that represent your relationship during each of these times. Don't think as you choose the symbols. Instead, work spontaneously, cutting out anything that impresses you and gluing it onto the collage in the appropriate section.

The goal of this exercise is not art, but collaborative expression. This is a chance for you to share how you see your relationship over time, without having to form the words yourself. You may want to add items with texture to the collage. For example, one woman with breast cancer glued her hospital bracelet directly in the middle of the collage.

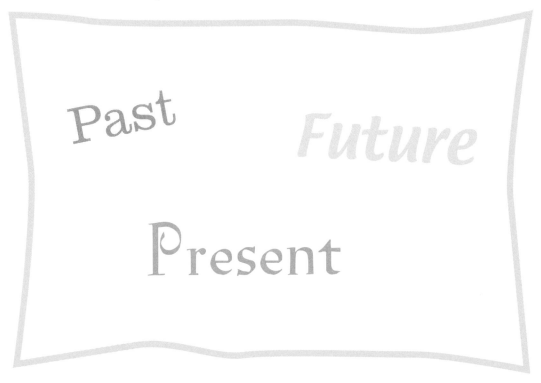

Touch, Sight, Sound, Smell, Taste— A Poem

For people with cancer and their partners, during and after treatment the senses seem at one time to be numb, at another to be terribly acute, but more often, bounce back and forth. Touching, for example, can seem desperately needed one day (by either partner) and on another day, very unwanted. But our senses—touch, sight, sound, smell, and taste—are very much a part of our responses to one another. So being aware of our senses and expressing how we are affected—in every sense—can help us to heal.

Writing poetry has traditionally been an effective way to express emotion. Some people believe that all poetry must rhyme. In fact, Robert Frost once said that writing a poem without using rhyme is like playing tennis without a net. But the experience of cancer teaches us that this disease sometimes doesn't come with a net, just as all our words do not fall into place in perfect rhyme. So we encourage free verse or rhymed verse for this exercise. The choice is yours. Write something—about the meaning of cancer, about its effect on each of your senses, or about its effect on your relationship—and share the poem with your partner. The poem doesn't need to be good or well written. The point is to express yourself freely.

The poem, *You and I,* by Donna Jones on the next page is an example of one woman's free expression using poetry.

You and I

by Donna Jones

You: with your ray-ravished throat
    tears and pain the only things
    you could swallow;
and I: unable to touch your hurt
    kissing the top of your head
    intoning the Oral Roberts mantra,
    "Heal! Heal!"

You: folded in on yourself lying on a cot;
    feeling, (you whisper),
    "like a wounded animal";
and I: coiled tightly on my side of the bed
    needing you, willing you
    curled warmly around me.

You: ringing the "I need help" bell,
    mouthing "I'm sorry"
    when I hurry to you;
and I: shocked awake from dreaming
    you whistling as once you did
    but assuring you,
    "It's all right; I'm right here."

You: one day rallying briefly
    to touch my hand
    and murmur my name
and I: filled at least
    for this moment
    with hope's
    most healing elixir:

You
and I…

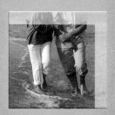

Resource Guide

Family Support and Services

AirLifeLine

50 Fullerton Court, Suite 200
Sacramento, CA 95825
Toll-free: 877-AIR-LIFE (877-247-5433)
Fax: 916-641-0600
Web site: *http://www.airlifeline.org*

Description: This nonprofit organization
provides free flights to patients who cannot
afford the cost of commercial airfare when
traveling to their medical facility.
AirLifeLine and the American Cancer
Society have formed a partnership with the
goal of making people across the United
States aware of this transportation service.

AMC Cancer Research Center & Foundation

1600 Pierce Street
Denver, CO 80214
Toll-free: 800-525-3777 (for cancer infor-
mation and counseling line)
Toll-free: 800-321-1557
Phone: 303-233-6501
Fax: 303-239-3340
Web site: *http://www.amc.org*

Description: Through the toll-free counseling line of this nonprofit research center, people can request free publications
and receive answers to questions about
cancer. The web site contains a section
about ongoing research and general information about specific types of cancer.

Cancer Care, Inc.

275 Seventh Avenue
New York, NY 10001
Toll-free: 800-813-HOPE (800-813-4673)
(for counseling)
Phone: 212-712-8080
Fax: 212-712-8495
Web site: *http://www.cancercare.org*
Web site (Spanish version):
http://www.cancercare.org/spanishmenu.htm

Description: A nonprofit social service
agency, Cancer Care, Inc. provides counseling and guidance to help people with
cancer, their families, and friends cope with
the impact of cancer. The web site includes
detailed information on specific cancers
and cancer treatment, clinical trials, and
links to other sites. The organization also

provides videos, support groups (online, telephone, and face-to-face), workshops, seminars and clinics, a newsletter, and other publications to interested consumers. *Spanish speaking staff is also available.*

Centering Corporation

7230 Maple Street
Omaha, NE 68134
Phone: 402-553-1200
Fax: 402-553-0507
Web site: *http://www.centering.org*

Description: The Centering Corporation is a nonprofit bereavement resource center. It provides books as well as audio and video materials for all age groups on a wide range of bereavement topics. Call to obtain a free catalog that lists over 300 resources, or access their web site for information on children and grief, infant loss, and the death of a child.

The Compassionate Friends

National Headquarters
P.O. Box 3696
Oak Brook, IL 60522-3696
Toll-free: 877-969-0010
Phone: 630-990-0010
Fax: 630-990-0246
Web site: *http://www.compassionatefriends.org*

Description: The Compassionate Friends is a nationwide self-help organization offering support to families who have experienced the death of a child, of any age, from any cause. It publishes a newsletter and other materials on parent and sibling bereavement. It makes referrals to nearly 600 local chapters.

The Dougy Center, The National Center for Grieving Children and Families

P.O. Box 86852
Portland, OR 97286
Phone: 503-775-5683
Fax: 503-777-3097
Web site: *http://www.grievingchild.org*

Description: The Dougy Center is a nonprofit support center that was founded in 1982 to help grieving children, teens, and families. They offer support and training locally, nationally, and internationally to individuals and organizations seeking to assist children and teens in grief.

Gilda's Club

322 Eighth Avenue, Suite 1402
New York, NY 10001
Toll-free: 888-GILDA 4 U (888-445-3248)
Phone: 917-305-1200
Fax: 917-305-0549
Web site: *http://www.gildasclub.org*

Description: Gilda's Club is a nonprofit organization providing a place where people with cancer and their families and friends join with others to build social and emotional support as a supplement to medical care. Services are free of charge and include support and networking groups, lectures and workshops, and social events. They offer a program called "Noogieland" for children with cancer and children whose parents have cancer.

Kids Konnected

27071 Cabot Road, Suite 102
Laguna Hills, CA 92653
Toll-free: 800-899-2866
Phone: 949-582-5443
Fax: 949-582-3983
Web site: *http://www.kidskonnected.org*

Description: Kids Konnected is a national, nonprofit organization that offers groups and programs for children who have a parent diagnosed with cancer. They provide answers to questions about cancer, support for children with a parent affected by cancer, an information packet with books and information specific to the needs of each child, referrals to local groups with monthly meetings, a quarterly newsletter for children, summer camps, socials, and grief workshops. They also have a program called "Teddy

Bear Outreach," which is designed to help young children after a parent has been diagnosed.

Hospice Net

401 Bowling Avenue, Suite 51
Nashville, TN 37205-5124
Web site: *http://www.hospicenet.org*

Description: Hospice Net is an independent nonprofit organization that works exclusively through the Internet. It contains more than one hundred articles regarding end-of-life issues. Hospice nurses, social workers, bereavement counselors, and chaplains are available to answer questions via e-mail. The web site includes information for patients and caregivers about hospice care, information about grief and loss, and a hospice locator service.

I Can Cope®

American Cancer Society (ACS)
Toll-free: 800-ACS-2345
Web site: *www.cancer.org*

Description: This program addresses the educational and psychological needs of people with cancer and their families. A series of eight classes discusses the disease, coping with daily health problems, controlling cancer-related pain, nutrition for the person with cancer, expressing feelings, living with limitations, and local resources. Through lectures, group discussions, and study assignments, the course helps people with cancer regain a sense of control over their lives.

Leukemia & Lymphoma Society (LLS)

1311 Mamaroneck Avenue
White Plains, NY 10605
Toll-free: 800-955-4572 (for the Information Resource Center)
Phone: 914-949-5213
Fax: 914-949-6691
Web site: *http://www.leukemia-lymphoma.org*

Description: The LLS is a national voluntary health agency dedicated to curing leukemia, lymphoma, Hodgkin's disease, and myeloma, and improving the quality of life of patients and their families. This organization was formerly known as the Leukemia Society of America (LSA). Patient service programs and resources available through local chapters of the LLS include financial assistance, support groups, one-to-one volunteer visitors (in some chapters), patient education and information, and referral to local resources in the community.

Look Good...Feel Better (LGFB)

American Cancer Society (ACS)
Cosmetic, Toiletry, and Fragrance Association Foundation (CTFA)
National Cosmetology Association (NCA)
Toll-free: 800-395-LOOK
Web site: *http://www.lookgoodfeelbetter.org*
Web site (Spanish version): *http://www.lookgoodfeelbetter.org/index_7.00.html*

Description: In partnership with the CTFA, the NCA, and the ACS, this free public service program is designed to teach women with cancer beauty techniques to help restore their appearance and self-image during chemotherapy and radiation treatment. *Information is also available in Spanish.*

Make Today Count

Mid-America Cancer Center
1235 East Cherokee
Springfield, MO 65804-2263
Toll-free: 800-432-2273
Phone: 417-885-2273
Fax: 417-888-8761

Description: Make Today Count is a nationwide support organization for people affected by cancer or other life-threatening illnesses. Its purpose is to enable individuals to cope with illness in a positive way by sharing experiences, coping skills, strength, and hope. Social workers provide telephone support, clearinghouse information, and referrals to chapters located throughout the United States.

Man to Man®

American Cancer Society (ACS)
Toll-free: 800-ACS-2345
Web site: *http://www.cancer.org*

Description: Man to Man is a prostate cancer education and support program that offers community-based group education, discussion, and support to men with prostate cancer.

National Association for Home Care (NAHC)

228 Seventh Street SE
Washington, DC 20003
Phone: 202-547-7424
Fax: 202-547-3540
Web site: *http://www.nahc.org*

Description: NAHC is a professional trade organization that represents more than 6,000 home care agencies, hospices, and home care aide organizations. It promotes and advocates for home care and hospice services, disseminates news and information, and provides a home care and hospice agency locator.

National Coalition for Cancer Survivorship (NCCS)

1010 Wayne Avenue, Suite 770
Silver Spring, MD 20910-5600
Toll-free: 877-NCCS-YES (877-622-7937) (for general information and publication orders)
Phone: 301-650-9127
Fax: 301-565-9670
Web site: *http://www.cansearch.org*

Description: The NCCS is a network of independent organizations working in the area of cancer survivorship and support. The web site offers links to online cancer resources, support groups, survivorship programs, the Cancer Survival Toolbox™, and newsletter.

National Family Caregivers Association (NFCA)

10400 Connecticut Avenue, #500
Kensington, MD 20895-3944
Toll-free: 800-896-3650
Phone: 301-942-6430
Fax: 301-942-2302
Web site: *http://www.nfcacares.org*

Description: NFCA is a national organization that focuses on family caregivers. It offers information and education, support, public awareness, and advocacy.

National Hospice and Palliative Care Organization (NHPCO)

1700 Diagonal Road, Suite 625
Alexandria, VA 22314
Toll-free: 800-658-8898 (for the Hospice Helpline)
Phone: 703-837-1500
Fax: 703-837-1233
Web site: *http://www.nhpco.org*

Description: NHPCO is a nonprofit, membership organization representing hospice and palliative care programs and professionals in the United States. The organization is committed to improving end of life care and expanding access to hospice care with the goal of enhancing the quality of life for people dying and their loved ones. The web site provides information about hospice programs in local areas and other publications.

National Lymphedema Network (NLN)

Latham Square
1611 Telegraph Avenue, Suite 1111
Oakland, CA 94612-2138
Toll-free: 800-541-3259 (for recorded information)
Phone: 510-208-3200

Fax: 510-208-3110

Web site: *http://www.lymphnet.org*

Description: The NLN is a nonprofit organization providing assistance to lymphedema patients, health care professionals, and the public by dissemination information on the prevention and management of lymphedema. *Some information is available in Spanish.*

Pharmaceutical Research and Manufacturers of America (PhRMA)

1100 Fifteenth Street NW, Suite 900
Washington, DC 20005
Phone: 202-835-3400
Fax: 202-835-3414
Web site: *http://www.phrma.org*

Description: This organization provides a *Directory of Prescription Drug Patient Assistance Programs* that contains information about how to make a request for assistance, what prescription medicines are covered, and basic eligibility criteria.

Reach to Recovery®

American Cancer Society (ACS)
Toll-free: 800-ACS-2345
Web site: *http://www.cancer.org*

Description: This program is designed to help patients with breast cancer cope with their diagnosis, treatment, and recovery. The volunteers in this program are women who have had breast cancer and are specially trained to share their knowledge and experiences in a supportive and nonintrusive manner. Ongoing support groups are available to help deal with the challenges of breast cancer. Reach to Recovery also provides early support to women who may have breast cancer or have just been diagnosed with cancer.

Visiting Nurse Associations of America (VNAA)

11 Beacon Street, Suite 910
Boston, MA 02108

Toll-free: 888-866-8773 or 800-426-2547
Phone: 617-523-4042
Fax: 617-227-4843
Web site: *http://www.vnaa.org*

Description: VNAA provides services including skilled nursing and mental health care, hospice care, and home health care.

Well Spouse Foundation

P.O. Box 30093
Elkins Park, PA 19027
Toll-free: 800-838-0879
Phone: 631-661-0421
Web site: *http://www.wellspouse.org*

Description: The Well Spouse Foundation is a national, nonprofit organization that provides support to partners of the chronically ill and/or disabled. They offer letter writing support groups, a bimonthly newsletter, annual conferences, and weekend meetings. They also make referrals to local support groups throughout the country. The organization is involved with other groups in educating health care professionals, politicians, and the public about the needs of "well spouses" and the importance of long-term care.

Wellness Community

35 East Seventh Street, Suite 412
Cincinnati, OH 45202-2420
Toll-free: 888-793-WELL (888-793-9355)
Phone: 513-421-7111
Fax: 513-421-7119
Web site: *http://www.thewellnesscommunity.org*

Description: The Wellness Community is a nonprofit organization whose mission is to help people with cancer and their families enhance their health and well-being by providing a professional program of emotional support, education, and hope. Support groups are facilitated by licensed counselors. Bereavement support groups are also available. Referrals are provided to their twenty-five facilities across the nation. The web site

has information about relaxation, talking
with children when a parent has cancer,
and an online support group for women
with breast cancer.

Y-ME National Breast Cancer Organization

212 West Van Buren, Suite 500
Chicago, IL 60607
Toll-free hotline: 800-221-2141
Toll-free hotline (Spanish): 800-986-9505
Phone: 312-986-8338
Fax: 312-294-8598

Web site: *http://www.y-me.org*
Web site (Spanish version): *http://www.y-me.org/spanish.htm*

Description: This organization focuses on
providing information and support to people
with breast cancer and their families. Y-ME
provides a national hotline, public meetings
and seminars, workshops for professionals,
referral services, support groups, a newsletter,
a resource library, a teen program, and
advocacy information. *Information is also
available in Spanish.*

Professional Mental Health Organizations

American Association for Marriage and Family Therapy (AAMFT)

1133 Fifteenth Street NW, Suite 300
Washington, DC 20005-2710
Phone: 202-452-0109
Fax: 202-223-2329
Web site: *http://www.aamft.org*

Description: This organization provides
referrals to local marriage and family
therapists. They also provide educational
materials on helping couples live with
illness and other issues related to families
and health.

American Association of Pastoral Counselors

9504A Lee Highway
Fairfax, VA 22031-2303
Toll-free: 800-225-5603
Phone: 703-385-6967
Fax: 703-352-7725
Web site: *http://www.aapc.org*

Description: This organization provides an
online directory of Certified Pastoral
Counselors across the country.

American Association of Sex Educators, Counselors and Therapists (AASECT)

P.O. Box 5488
Richmond, VA 23220
Web site: *http://www.aasect.org*

Description: AASECT is a nonprofit,
interdisciplinary professional organization.
In addition to sex educators, sex counselors,
and sex therapists, AASECT members
include physicians, nurses, social workers,
psychologists, allied health professionals,
clergy members, lawyers, sociologists,
marriage and family planning specialists,
and researchers, as well as students in
relevant professional disciplines. Members
share an interest in promoting understanding of human sexuality and healthy sexual
behavior.

AASECT can provide a list of AASECT-certified counselors and/or therapists. To obtain a list, send a stamped, self-addressed business-size envelope to the above address.

American Counseling Association (ACA)

5999 Stevenson Avenue
Alexandria, VA 22304-3300
Toll-free: 800-347-6647
Phone: 703-823-9800
Fax: 703-823-0252
Web site: *http://www.counseling.org*

Description: The ACA provides information in the field of counseling and public fact sheets on coping with crisis.

American Psychiatric Association

1400 K Street NW
Washington, DC 20005
Toll-free: 888-357-7924
Fax: 202-682-6850
Web site: *http://www.psych.org*

Description: This organization provides information on mental health and referrals.

American Psychological Association (APA)

750 First Street NE
Washington, DC 20002-4242
Toll-free: 800-374-2721
Phone: 202-336-5500
Phone (TDD/TTY): 202-336-6123
Fax: 202-336-5997
Web site: *http://www.apa.org*

Description: The APA offers referrals to psychologists in local areas. They also provide information on family issues, parenting, and health. The APA web site has links to state psychological associations that may also provide local referrals.

International Society of Psychiatric-Mental Health Nurses (ISPN)

1211 Locust Street
Philadelphia, PA 19107
Toll-free: 800-826-2950
Phone: 215-545-2843
Fax: 215-545-8107
Web site: *http://www.ispn-psych.org*

Description: The ISPN consists of specialty psychiatric-mental health nurses who treat patients with medical and mental health issues through counseling and education.

National Association of Social Workers (NASW)

750 First Street NE, Suite 700
Washington, DC 20002-4241
Toll-free: 800-638-8799
Phone: 202-408-8600
Web site: *http://www.naswdc.org*

Description: This organization is concerned with advocacy, work practice standards and ethics, and professional standards for agencies employing social workers. The web site provides a national register of clinical social workers for local referrals.

National Board of Certified Counselors (NBCC)

3 Terrace Way, Suite D
Greensboro, NC 27403-3660
Phone: 336-547-0607
Fax: 336-547-0017
Web site: *http://www.nbcc.org*

Description: NBCC, an independent, nonprofit credentialing body for counselors, focuses on promoting quality counseling through certification. On their web site, they provide information about how to locate a professional counselor called *CounselorFind*.

Cancer Information

American Cancer Society (ACS)
Toll-free: 800-ACS-2345
Web site: *http://www.cancer.org*

Description: The ACS is the nationwide, community-based, voluntary health organization dedicated to eliminating cancer as a major health problem by preventing cancer, saving lives, and diminishing suffering from cancer through research, education, advocacy, and service. The ACS provides educational materials and information on cancer, maintains several patient programs, directs people to services in their community including workshops and support groups, and provides funding for research.

American Medical Association (AMA)
515 North State Street
Chicago, IL 60610
Toll-free: 800-621-8335 (for order placement)
Phone: 312-464-5000
Fax: 312-464-5600
Web site: *http://www.ama-assn.org*

Description: The AMA develops and promotes standards in medical practice, research, and education. Under the consumer health information section, the web site contains databases on physicians and hospitals that can be searched by medical specialty. A pull-down menu of specific conditions is also provided.

American Society for Therapeutic Radiology and Oncology (ASTRO)
12500 Fair Lakes Circle, Suite 375
Fairfax, VA 22033-3882
Toll-free: 800-962-7876
Phone: 703-502-1550
Fax: 703-502-7852
Web site: *http://www.astro.org*

Description: Focusing on the use of radiation therapy for the treatment of cancer, this society's web site includes an overview of radiation therapy and a list of frequently asked questions.

American Society of Clinical Oncology (ASCO)
1900 Duke Street, Suite 200
Alexandria, VA 22314
Toll-free: 888-651-3038 (Patient Services Hotline)
Phone: 703-299-0150
Fax: 703-299-1044
Web site: *http://www.asco.org*

Description: The ASCO is an international medical society representing about 10,000 cancer specialists involved in clinical research and patient care. The ASCO web site is a resource for cancer patients, doctors, and researchers and includes patient guides, a glossary of cancer terms, an ASCO member oncologist locator, news and information about different cancers and drug treatments, information about cancer legislation, summaries of government reports, and links to related sites.

Association of Community Cancer Centers (ACCC)
11600 Nebel Street, Suite 201
Rockville, MD 20852-2557
Fax: 301-770-1949
Web site: *http://www.accc-cancer.org*

Description: This national organization includes over 600 medical centers, hospitals, and cancer programs. The web site contains a searchable database of cancer centers listed by state, as well as information about oncology drugs (registration is required), and specific cancers.

Cancer Research Institute (CRI)

681 Fifth Avenue
New York, NY 10022
Toll-free: 800-99-CANCER (800-992-2623)
Phone: 212-688-7515
Fax: 212-832-9376
Web site: *http://www.cancerresearch.org*

Description: An institute funding cancer research and providing public information on cancer immunology and cancer treatment, the CRI helps locate immunotherapy clinical trials and offers a cancer reference guide and other informational booklets.

Centers for Disease Control and Prevention (CDC)

Public Inquiries/MASO
Mailstop F07
1600 Clifton Road NE
Atlanta, GA 30333
Phone: 404-639-3534
Toll-free: 800-311-3435
Web site: *http://www.cdc.gov*

Description: The CDC is an agency of the U.S. Department of Health and Human Services. Their mission is to promote health and quality of life by preventing and controlling disease, injury, and disability. Their web site contains a searchable map of centers, information about health topics, downloadable publications, and links to related sources.

Division of Cancer Prevention and Control (DCPC)

CDC/DCPC
4770 Buford Highway NE
Mailstop K64
Atlanta, GA 30341
Toll-free: 888-842-6355
Fax: 770-488-4760
Web site: *http://www.cdc.gov/cancer*

Description: The DCPC is within the National Center for Chronic Disease Prevention and Health Promotion. It conducts, supports, and promotes efforts to prevent cancer and to increase early detection of cancer. The DCPC works with partners in the government, private, and nonprofit sectors to develop, implement, and promote effective cancer prevention and control practices nationwide. The toll-free number can be used to locate free or low-cost mammography and Pap test centers in local areas. The web site contains a searchable map of centers, information about breast cancer, downloadable publications, and links to related sources.

MayoClinic.Com

Mayo Foundation for Medical Education and Research
First Street SW
Rochester, MN 55905
Web site: *http://www.mayoclinic.com*

Description: This web site contains a database searchable by keyword and topic. It also offers questions and answers from Mayo Clinic specialists, as well as links to reference articles and cancer organizations.

Medscape

Web site: *http://www.medscape.com*

Description: Although a no-cost registration is required to view some of the content, this web site offers a great deal of information on prescription drugs as well as medical articles. There are also links to several organizations, cancer centers, database and education web sites, journals, and government sites. The web site is searchable by keyword.

National Bone Marrow Transplant Link (NBMT Link)

20411 West 12 Mile Road, Suite 108
Southfield, MI 48076
Toll-free: 800-LINK-BMT (800-546-5268)
Phone: 248-358-1886
Fax: 248-358-1889
Web site: *http://www.nbmtlink.org*

Description: The NBMT Link is a non-profit organization that serves as an information center for prospective Bone Marrow Transplant (BMT) patients and as a resource for health professionals. NBMT Link provides peer support to BMT patients and their families over the telephone. The peer-support volunteers are BMT transplant survivors who have been specially trained. The web site has information for donors and transplant patients.

National Cancer Institute (NCI)

NCI Public Inquiries Office
Building 31, Room 10A31
31 Center Drive, MSC 2580
Bethesda, MD 20892-2580
Phone: 301-435-3848
Web site: *http://www.cancer.gov*
Web site (Spanish version):
http://www.cancer.gov/espanol

Description: This government agency under the National Institutes of Health (NIH) provides cancer information through several services (see list below). The Cancer Information Service's toll-free number provides accurate, up-to-date information about cancer to patients and their families, health professionals, and the general public.

Cancer Information Service (CIS)

Toll-free: 800-4-CANCER
(800-422-6237)
Toll-free (TTY): 800-322-8615
Web site: *http://www.cancer.gov/cancer_information*

Description: The CIS provides information to consumers and health care professionals. The web site contains a wealth of information including pamphlets and brochures on cancer diagnosis, treatment, research, and prevention. The NCI also maintains a listing of current clinical trials and other resources that may be helpful. The NCI can also

provide free pamphlets on various forms of cancer treatment, medication, clinical trials, and other cancer-related information. *Spanish speaking staff is available.*

CancerFax

Toll-free fax: 800-624-2511
Fax: 301-402-5874

Description: CancerFax contains PDQ® (Physician's Data Query) full-text summaries on cancer treatment, screening, prevention, genetics, and supportive care; fact sheets on current cancer topics; and topic searches from the CANCERLIT database. To obtain a contents list, dial the fax number and follow the recorded instructions.

CANCERLIT (Bibliographic Database)

Web site: *http://www.cancer.gov/cancer_information/cancer_literature*

Description: This searchable site contains cancer articles published in medical and scientific journals, books, government reports, and articles that were presented at national meetings.

CancerTrials

Web site: *http://www.cancer.gov/clinical_trials*

Description: This site offers information about ongoing cancer clinical trials and explanations of what a trial is and what is involved.

Physician Data Query (PDQ®)

Web site: *http://www.cancer.gov/cancer_information/pdq*

Description: PDQ is NCI's comprehensive cancer database. It contains peer-reviewed summaries on cancer treatment, screening, prevention, genetics, and supportive care. It also maintains a registry of cancer clinical trials from around the world, and directories of physicians, professionals who provide genetics services, and organizations that provide cancer care.

National Center for Complementary and Alternative Medicine (NCCAM)

NCCAM Clearinghouse
P.O. Box 7923
Gaithersburg, MD 20898
Toll-free: 888-644-6226
Toll-free (TTY): 866-464-3615
Phone: 301-519-3153
Toll-free fax: 866-464-3616
Web site: *http://nccam.nih.gov*

Description: This NIH web site provides information on some complementary and alternative methods being promoted to treat different diseases. Many of NCCAM's resources are also available on the NCCAM web site.

National Comprehensive Cancer Network (NCCN)

50 Huntingdon Pike, Suite 200
Rockledge, PA 19046
Toll-free: 800-909-NCCN (800-909-6226)
Phone: 215-728-4788
Fax: 215-728-3877
Web site: *http://www.nccn.org*

Description: The NCCN is a nonprofit organization that is an alliance of cancer centers. The American Cancer Society (ACS) has partnered with NCCN to translate the *NCCN Clinical Practice Guidelines* into a patient-friendly resource. The guidelines offer easy to understand information for patients and family members about treatment options for each stage of cancer. The treatment guidelines for patients are available for breast, prostate, lung, colon and rectal cancer, nausea and vomiting, fever and neutropenia, cancer-related fatigue, and cancer pain. More guidelines are currently being developed. Call the ACS for the latest guidelines or

view them online at either www.cancer.org or www.nccn.org. *Guidelines are also available in Spanish.*

National Library of Medicine (includes MEDLINE)

8600 Rockville Pike
Bethesda, MD 20894
Toll-free: 888-FIND-NLM (888-346-3656) (Reference and Customer Service Desk)
Phone: 301-594-5983 (for local and international calls)
Fax: 301-402-1384
Web site: *http://www.nlm.nih.gov*

Description: This NIH web site provides a search engine for health, medical, and scientific literature and research, as well as links to other government resources.

NLM Gateway

Web site: *http://gateway.nlm.nih.gov/ gw/Cmd*

Description: As part of the National Library of Medicine (NLM), this web site offers links to searchable databases and allows users to search simultaneously in multiple retrieval systems at the NLM.

PubMed

Web site: *http://www.ncbi.nlm.nih.gov/ PubMed*

Description: Also part of the NLM, this web site provides access to literature references in MEDLINE and other databases, with links to online journals. The site is searchable by keyword.

National Women's Health Information Center (NWHIC)

The Office on Women's Health
U.S. Department of Health and Human Services
8550 Arlington Boulevard, Suite 300
Fairfax, VA 22301
Toll-free: 800-994-WOMAN (800-994-9662)

Toll-free (TDD): 888-220-5446
Phone: 703-560-6618
Fax: 703-560-6598
Web site: *http://www.4woman.gov*
Web site (Spanish version):
http://www.4woman.gov/Spanish

Description: This web site has a searchable database of information on various women's health issues, including breast cancer. Documents accessible through this site include information from the NCI, the CDC, and several other government agencies. The site contains a section for special groups, which separates breast cancer and other health information by specific minority group. It also contains links to online medical dictionaries and journals. *Spanish speaking staff and materials are available.*

OncoLink

OncoLink Editorial Board
University of Pennsylvania Cancer Center
3400 Spruce Street - 2 Donner
Philadelphia, PA 19104-4283
Fax: 215-349-5445
Web site: *http://www.oncolink.com*

Description: OncoLink is a service provided by the University of Pennsylvania and the University of Pennsylvania Cancer Center. Its mission is to help cancer patients, families, health care professionals, and the general public get accurate cancer-related information free of charge. The web site provides information on cancer including clinical trials, support groups, educational materials, cancer screening and prevention, financial questions, and other resources for people with cancer.

SHARE–Self-Help for Women with Breast or Ovarian Cancer

1501 Broadway, Suite 1720
New York, NY 10036
Toll-free: 866-891-2392
Phone (Breast Cancer Hotline):
212-382-2111
Phone (Ovarian Cancer Hotline):
212-719-1204
Phone (Spanish Hotline): 212-719-4454
Phone (Business Office): 212-719-0364
Fax: 212-869-3431
Web site: *http://www.sharecancersupport.org*

Description: SHARE is a self-help organization that serves women who have been affected by breast or ovarian cancer. Hotline volunteers are breast or ovarian cancer survivors. They provide information about cancer, emotional support, printed materials, and referrals to national organizations. Their web site includes information on the hotlines and support programs in New York City. *Spanish speaking staff available.*

Additional Reading

Pamphlets

After Diagnosis: A Guide for Patients and Families. Atlanta, Ga.: American Cancer Society, 800-ACS-2345 (www.cancer.org).

How to Find a Financial Professional Sensitive to Cancer Issues. Atlanta, Ga.: American Cancer Society, 800-ACS-2345 (www.cancer.org).

It Helps to Have Friends When Mom or Dad Has Cancer. Atlanta, Ga.: American Cancer Society, 800-ACS-2345 (www.cancer.org).

Sexuality and Cancer: For the Man Who Has Cancer and His Partner. Atlanta, Ga.: American Cancer Society, 800-ACS-2345 (www.cancer.org).

Sexuality and Cancer: For the Woman Who Has Cancer and Her Partner. Atlanta, Ga.: American Cancer Society, 800-ACS-2345 (www.cancer.org).

When Someone in Your Family Has Cancer. Bethesda, Md.: National Cancer Institute, 800-4-CANCER (www.cancer.gov).

Books

Ackermann, A., and A. Ackermann. 2002. *Our Mom Has Cancer.* Atlanta, Ga.: American Cancer Society.

American Cancer Society. 2001. *A Breast Cancer Journey.* Atlanta, Ga.: American Cancer Society.

American Cancer Society. 2002. *American Cancer Society's Complementary and Alternative Cancer Methods Handbook.* Atlanta, Ga.: American Cancer Society.

American Cancer Society. 2000. *American Cancer Society's Guide to Complementary and Alternative Cancer Methods.* Atlanta, Ga.: American Cancer Society.

American Cancer Society. 2001. *American Cancer Society's Guide to Pain Control.* Atlanta, Ga.: American Cancer Society.

American Cancer Society. 2002. *Because… Someone I Love Has Cancer: Kids' Activity Book.* Atlanta, Ga.: American Cancer Society.

American Cancer Society. 2001. *Cancer in the Family: Helping Children Cope with a Parent's Illness.* Atlanta, Ga.: American Cancer Society.

American Cancer Society. 2002. *Crossing Divides: A Couple's Story of Cancer, Hope, and Hiking Montana's Continental Divide.* Atlanta, Ga.: American Cancer Society.

Bostwick, D. G., G. T. MacLennan, and T. R. Larson. 1999. *Prostate Cancer: What Every Man—and His Family—Needs to Know.* Rev. ed. New York: Villard.

Davis, M., M. McKay, and E. R. Eshelman. 2000. *Relaxation and Stress Reduction Workbook.* Oakland, Ca.: New Harbinger Publications.

Eyre, H. J., D. P. Lange, and L. B. Morris. 2001. *Informed Decisions: The Complete Book of Cancer Diagnosis, Treatment, and Recovery, Second ed.* Atlanta, Ga.: American Cancer Society.

Gottman, J. and J. Declair. 2001. *The Relationship Cure: A Five-Step Guide for Building Better Connections with Family, Friends, and Lovers.* New York: Crown Publishing Group (Random House).

Gray, J. 1992. *Men are From Mars, Women are From Venus: A Practical Guide for Improving Communication and Getting What You Want in Your Relationships.* New York: HarperCollins.

Harpham, W. S. 1997. *When a Parent Has Cancer: A Guide to Caring for Your Children.* New York: HarperCollins.

Hendrix, H. 2001. *Getting the Love You Want: A Guide for Couples.* New York: Owl Books (Henry Holt and Company).

Holland, J. C., and S. Lewis. 2000. *The Human Side of Cancer: Living with Hope, Coping with Uncertainty.* New York: HarperCollins.

Houts, P., and J. Bucher. 2000. *Caregiving: A Step-By-Step Resource for Caring for the Person with Cancer at Home.* Atlanta, Ga.: American Cancer Society.

Laughlin, E. H. 2001. *Coming to Terms with Cancer: A Glossary of Cancer-Related Terms.* Atlanta, Ga.: American Cancer Society.

Levin, B. 1999. *Colorectal Cancer: A Thorough and Compassionate Resource for Patients and Their Families.* New York: Villard.

McCue, K. 1996. *How to Help Children Through a Parent's Serious Illness.* Third ed. New York: St. Martin's Press.

McGraw, P. 2001. *Dr. Phil Getting Real: Lessons in Life, Marriage, and Family.* Carlsbad, Ca.: Hay House, Inc.

McKay, M., P. Fanning, and K. Paleg. 1994. *Couple Skills: Making Your Relationship Work.* Oakland, Ca.: New Harbinger Publications, Inc.

National Family Caregivers Association. 1996. *The Resourceful Caregiver: Helping Family Caregivers Help Themselves.* St. Louis: Mosby Lifeline (Times Mirror Company).

Runowicz, C. D., J. A. Petrek, and T. S. Gansler. 1999. *Women and Cancer: A Thorough and Compassionate Resource for Patients and Their Families.* New York: Villard.

Schover, L. 1997. *Sexuality and Fertility After Cancer.* New York: John Wiley and Sons.

Tannen, D. 2001. *You Just Don't Understand: Women and Men in Conversation.* New York: Quill (HarperCollins).

Wallerstein, J., and S. Blakeslee. 1996. *The Good Marriage: How and Why Love Lasts.* New York: Warner Books.

Wilkes, G. M., T. B. Ades, and I. Krakoff. 2000. *Consumers Guide to Cancer Drugs.* Sudbury, Maine: Jones and Bartlett.

A

A Collage of Pictures and Words, 242

acquired immunodeficiency syndrome
  (AIDS), 15–16

active ingredients of couples' relationships, 42–58

adoptions, 89, 179

affairs, extramarital, 93–96, 180–182

Al-Anon, 188

alcohol, 12, 83, 99
  and drug abuse, 105–108, 187–190

all or none thinking, 134–135

American Association of Sex Educators,
  Counselors and Therapists
  (AASECT), 173, 250–251

anger
  after treatment, 6–7
  caregiver, 29, 35
  and communication, 65–66, 131–132
  and couples therapy, 197
  and diagnosis, 5, 13
  effects on relationships, 81–82

anxiety, 15, 36, 210
  about sex, 163–166

attachment, 44–51

B

banking sperm, eggs, and embryos, 177

behavioral therapy, 200–201

bladder cancer, 13

Blakeslee, Sandra, 61–62

blended families, 120–122, 190–191

body image, 165

body language, 138

brain tumors, 11

breast cancer, 8, 14–15, 73, 160

brief therapy, 204

burnout, caregiver, 33–35

C

Can Cancer Be Funny?, 233

cancer
  bladder, 13
  blood system, 15, 177, 190
  brain, 11
  breast, 8, 14–15, 73, 160
  diagnosis, 4–5
  effects on both partners, xiii–xiv, 3–7,
    213
  female, 14–15
  gastrointestinal, 12–13
  head and neck, 11–12
  HIV-related, 15–16
  lung, 13
  male, 14, 177
  prostate, 14
  testicular, 14, 177
  treatment, 5–7
  understanding, 10

caregivers
  and adjusting to changes in the
    patient, 28–29
  burnout, 33–35
  and communicating with children,
    24–26
  communication tips for, 30–31, 143

coordinating care, 26–27
and delegation, 34
and depression, 36, 78
and emotional health care, 36
feelings of, 21–23, 35–36, 78
and gender, 8
guilt, 29, 33
and obtaining information, 23
positive aspects for, 37
and role changes, 16–17
and stress, 7–9
taking care of, 31–33, 142, 192
tasks of, 23–28, 235
types of support services for, 27–28
and workplace issues, 24
catharsis approach to conflict, 82–83
cervical cancer, 14
children
adopting, 89, 110, 179
answering difficult questions from,
115–117
and attachment, 44–45
and balancing needs as a couple,
63–64, 109–110
in blended families, 120–122, 191
communicating with, 24–26, 111–117
coping strategies for, 117–119
and discipline, 119
of divorced parents, 97–98, 183
of dual-career couples, 123
maintaining normal routines for, 26,
118–119
and overcoming infertility, 13, 15,
88–89, 175–179
and parenting styles, 110
Circles of Feeling, 218–221
cognitive distortions, 132–137, 200–201
cold shoulder approach to conflict, 82
commitment, 43–44, 62, 197
communication
about death, 237
about needs and emotions, 22–23,
235–237

about sexuality, 240–241
about spirituality, 238
and all or none thinking, 134–135
and asking for things one needs,
138–139, 234–235
and body language, 138
building basic skills in, 130–131
with children about cancer, 24–26,
111–117
and cognitive distortions, 132–137
and control fallacies, 136
and core arguments, 142
and couples therapy, 197
and criticism, 54, 239
and expressing feelings, 136–139
and fractured logic, 135–136
and gender, 56–57
and global labeling, 135
and Learning to Listen, 214–217, 221,
229, 230
and magnification, 134
and mind reading, 133
open, 65–67
politeness in, 132
problems, 52–53, 129–130, 198,
224–229
and reasons for conflict, 53–54
and Runners and Chasers, 224–229
and sexual intimacy, 160
therapies, 203
and Three to One, 239
tips for caregivers, 30–31, 35, 143
and tunnel vision, 133–134
and ways to resolve conflicts,
139–144
why and how to engage in, 51–53
compromise, 140–141
conflicts, relationship, 18, 53–54
and compromise, 140–141
and core arguments, 91–93, 142
and divorce, 96–98
and domestic violence, 98–105
and empathy, 131

and extramarital affairs, 93–96
and problem solving steps, 141–142
and Runner and Chasers, 224–229
styles, 82–84, 224–229
ways to resolve, 139–144
confusion and memory loss
and brain tumors, 11
and HIV-related cancers, 15–16
connection, 44–51
control fallacies, 136
coordination of care, 26–27
coping strategies
for children of patients, 117–119
and common dilemmas, 16–18
and depression, 79
for difficult feelings, 221
and disruption of routines, 17
and effects on both partners, 6–7
and long-term planning, 17–18
and personal responsibility, 19
and relationship conflicts, 18
and religion, 19
and role changes, 16–17
role of ethnicity and culture in, 18–19
and styles, 16
core arguments between partners, 91–93,
142
couples
and active ingredients of relationships, 42–58
and blended families, 120–122,
190–191
and children, 63–64, 175–179
and Circles of Feeling, 218–221
and commitment, 43–44, 62
common dilemmas faced by, 16–18
and communication, 51–57, 65–67,
214–217, 224–229
and conflict styles, 82–84, 224–229
and connection, 44–51
coping styles of, 16
and criticism, 54, 239
differences in, xii–xiii

and discussions about death, 235
and divorce, 96–98, 182–184
and domestic violence, 98–105,
184–187
dual-career, 122–124, 192–193
effects of cancer on, 7–9, 213
and empathy, 130–131
and evaluating relationships, 59
and exploring strengths and problems,
48–49
and extramarital affairs, 93–96,
180–182
fears, communicating and managing,
230–231
and gender differences, 56–57
and ghosts from the past, 150–151
and improving relationships, 69–70
and independence, 50–51, 62–63
and individual needs, 43–44, 142,
192, 198
and laughter, 68, 154, 233
and Learning to Listen, 214–217, 221,
229, 230
negotiating skills for, 232
and nurturing love, 151–153, 216
pictures of, 216–217, 242
and power struggles, 84
remarried, 190–191
and the role of ethnicity and culture
in coping, 18–19
same-sex, 124–125, 193–194
and sexual intimacy, 57–58, 67–68,
240–241
and sharing crises, 64–65
signs of trouble in, 198–199
therapy, 195–206
three phases of relationships in,
41–42, 69–70
and unassertive partners, 54–56
uniqueness of the bond in, 39–41
working as a team, 155–156
Couples' Corner workbook, 213–244
and asking for help, 235

and childhood memories, 222–223
and Circles of Feeling, 218–221
and discussing death, 237
and fears, 230–231
and humor, 233
and journaling, 216–217, 233
and Learning to Listen, 214–217, 229, 230
and Let's Make a Deal, 232
and Our Support, 234
and pictures, 216–217, 242
and poetry, 243–244
purpose of, 213
and Runners and Chasers, 224–229
and sexuality, 240–241
and Simple Pleasures, 236
and spirituality, 238
and Three to One, 239
courtesy, 132
crises, sharing, 64–65, 95, 198
criticism, 54, 239
cycle of violence, 101–102

D
death, 237
delegation, 34
depression, 5, 15, 210
    caregiver, 36, 78
    defining, 78–81
    and divorce, 97
    effects on relationships, 77–81
    professional help for, 81
    symptoms of, 79–80
    treatment for, 80
Desire Diary, 163
diagnosis
    effects on both partners, 4–5
    effects on caregivers, 21–22
    initial reactions to, 10, 21–22
differentiation, 202
discrimination, against same-sex couples, 124–125
disruption of routines, 17

and children, 26, 118–119
divorce, xiii, 96–98, 182–184
domestic violence, 98–105, 184–187
drug abuse, 105–108
dual-career couples, 122–124, 192–193

E
Ellison, Carol, 57
emotions (*See also* Intimacy, emotional)
    and addressing upsetting thoughts, 169–171
    of anger, 5–7, 29, 35, 65–66, 81–82
    of caregivers, 21–23, 35
    and childhood memories, 222–223
    and Circles of Feeling, 218–221
    and communication styles, 51–52, 65–67
    of depression, 5, 15, 36, 77–81
    and diagnosis, 4–5
    and emotional health care, 36
    expressing, 136–139
    and fear of abuse or rejection, 48
    and honesty, 148–150, 180
    of love, 151–153
    and poetry, 243–244
    problems with showing, 85–86
    and self-acceptance, 145–148
    and sexual intimacy, 57–58, 241–242
    and Simple Pleasures, 236
    and ways to resolve conflicts, 139–144
empathy, 130–131
escape approach to conflict, 83–84
ethnicity and culture and coping styles, 18–19
extramarital affairs, 93–96, 180–182

F
family systems therapy, 202
fatigue, 5, 13
fears
    of abuse or rejection, 47–48
    of caregivers, 30–31, 35

of children of patients, 117
common, 4
communicating and managing, 230–231
and honesty, 149–150
female cancers, 14–15
financial costs, 9
of couples therapy, 204–206
fractured logic, 135–136
Frost, Robert, 243

G
gastrointestinal cancer, 12–13
gender
and communication styles, 56–57
and effects of cancer on healthy partners, 8
Getting the Most from Sex, 240–241
global labeling, 135
Good Marriage: How & Why Love Lasts, The, 61
Gray, John, 56
guilt
caregiver, 12–13, 29, 33
children feeling, 119
and domestic violence, 186
patient, 4–5, 12–13
gynecological cancers, 14

H
HIV-related cancers, 15–16
honesty, 148–150, 180
hospitalization, effects on both partners, 5–6
human immunodeficiency virus (HIV), 15–16
human papilloma virus, 14
humor, 68, 154, 233

I
impotence, 13, 14
incontinence, 14
independence, 50–51, 62–63, 235

individual therapy, 209–211
infertility, 13, 15, 88–89, 175–177
solutions for, 177–179
information
and burnout, 34
giving children, 24–26
obtaining, 23
and sexual intimacy, 160
intimacy
emotional (*See also* Emotions)
and nurturing love, 151–153
removing obstacles to, 156–157
through honesty, 148–150
through self-acceptance, 145–148
through spirituality, 154–155
and working as a team, 155–156
physical (*See* Sexual intimacy)

J
journaling, 216, 233
Just from You, 235

L
laughter, 68, 154, 233
Learning to Listen, 214–217, 221, 229, 230
Lesko, Lynna, 4
Let's Make a Deal, 232
leukemias and lymphomas, 15, 177, 190
long-term planning, 6, 17–18
love, nurturing, 151–153, 216
lumpectomies, 14
lung cancer, 13

M
magnification, 134
male cancers, 14, 177
marital therapy, 195–206
marriage counseling, 195–206
masturbation, 164
memories, childhood, 222–223
men
as caregivers, 8

and male cancers, 14, 177
Men Are from Mars, Women Are from Venus, 56
menopause, 14–15, 161
mind reading, 133
Must We Talk about Death?, 237

N
negotiation, 232
Northouse, Laurel, 8

O
obstacles to emotional intimacy, 156–157
Our Greatest Fears, 230–231
Our Support, 234
ovarian cancer, 14

P
pain during intercourse, 13, 171
patients
    adjusting to changes in, 28–29
    and asking for help from caregivers, 235
    coordinating care for, 26–27
    and discussions about death, 235
    initial reactions to diagnosis, 10
    and role changes, 16–17
    and Simple Pleasures, 236
    and understanding what they are experiencing, 10
    and workplace issues, 24
peer support groups, 207–208
personal responsibility
    and coping styles, 19
    and domestic abuse, 100–101
    for one's own needs, 142
phases of couples' relationships, 41–42
physical abuse, 98–100
physical appearance
    adjusting to changes in, 28–29, 160–162, 165
    and head and neck cancer, 11–12

and sexual intimacy, 87–88
pictures of couples, 216–217, 242
Pittman, Frank, 96
poetry, 243–244
politeness, 132
power struggles, 84
problem solving steps, 141–142
prostate cancer, 14
psychodynamic approaches to couples therapy, 201–202
psychological battering, 98
psychological impact
    of bladder cancer, 13
    of brain tumors, 11
    of breast cancer, 14–15, 73
    and communication, 30–31
    of female cancers, 14–15
    of gastrointestinal cancer, 12–13
    of head and neck cancer, 11–12
    of leukemias and lymphomas, 15
    of lung cancer, 13
    of male cancers, 14

Q
questions from the past, 49
Questions of Spirit, 238

R
radical cystectomies, 13
recurrence, fear of, 10
religion and spirituality
    building closeness through, 154–155
    and coping styles, 19
    discussing, 238
    and spiritual support, 35
remarried couples, 190–191
Resource Guide, 245–258
    Additional Reading, 257–258
    Cancer Information, 252–256
    Family Support and Services, 245–250
    Professional Mental Health Organizations, 250–251

role changes, 16–17
Runners and Chasers, 224–229

S
same-sex couples, 124–125, 193–194
self-acceptance, 145–148
self-esteem
    and domestic violence, 99, 104–105
    and infertility, 89
    and role changes, 17
sexual abuse, 98
sexual intimacy
    and addressing upsetting thoughts,
        169–171
    and bladder cancer, 13
    and changing the routine, 169
    and communication, 160, 240–241
    and coping with changes in appear-
        ance, 28–29, 87–88, 160–162,
        165
    and counseling, 171–173, 197
    and creativity, 168–169
    difficulties, 57–58, 86–88
    effect of cancer on, 159–160
    and extramarital affairs, 93–96
    and female cancers, 14–15
    and gastrointestinal cancer, 12–13
    and happiness, 67–68
    and imbalances in desire, 162–164
    and impotence, 12–13
    improving, 240–241
    and infertility, 13, 15, 88–89,
        177–179
    and male cancers, 14
    and masturbation, 164
    overcoming anxiety about, 163–166
    resuming, 166–168
    when to avoid, 170
silence and withdrawal, 82
Simple Pleasures, 236
six Ds, 4
smoking
    and head and neck cancer, 12

and lung cancer, 13
social costs, 9
spirituality (*See* Religion and spirituality)
Still Kids Together, 222–223
stomas, 12–13
stress
    and caregivers, 8
    coping with, xiii, 6, 8–9
    financial, 9
    and improving relationships, 69–70,
        189
    social, 9
suicide, 12, 81, 97
support services
    for caregivers, 34
    for children of patients, 118
    couples therapy, 195–206
    and Our Support, 234
    for same-sex couples, 194
    self-help, 207–208
    for sexual counseling, 171–173
    and therapy groups, 208–209
    types of, 27–28, 196
    when to seek, 196–198

T
Tannen, Deborah, 56–57
testicular cancer, 14, 177
Then and Now, 216–217
therapy, couples
    behavioral, 200–201
    brief, 204
    and choosing a therapist, 205
    communication, 203
    family systems, 202
    groups, 208–209
    how to pay for, 204–206
    and individual therapy, 209–211
    marriage or relationship enrichment,
        204
    psychodynamic approaches to,
        201–202
    reasons to start, 198–199

and self-help support groups, 207–208
specific approaches used in, 199–204
and support groups, 206–207
types of, 195–196
when to seek, 196–198
third party reproduction, 178
Three to One, 239
tobacco (*See* Smoking)
Touch, Sight, Sound, Smell, Taste—A
        Poem, 243–244
treatment
    for depression, 80
    effects on both partners, 5–7
triangles concept, 202
tunnel vision, 133–134

U
unassertive partners, 54–56
uterine cancer, 14

V
vaginal cancer, 14
verbal abuse, 100
victims of abuse, 104–105, 186–187

W
Walker, Lenore, 101
Wallerstein, Judith, 61–62
ways to share, 153
women
    and breast cancer, 8, 14–15
    as caregivers, 8
    and gynecological cancers, 14
workplace issues, 24, 193

Y
You Just Don't Understand: Women and
    Men in Conversation, 56–57

About the Authors

Joy L. Fincannon, R.N., M.S., is an Associate Medical Editor at the American Cancer Society in Atlanta, Georgia. She is a psychiatric clinical nurse specialist experienced in working with cancer patients, their families, and cancer health professionals. Ms. Fincannon has published in nursing journals and medical textbooks and has been a psychotherapist in private practice for many years.

Katherine V. Bruss, Psy.D., is the former Managing Editor for book publishing at the American Cancer Society in Atlanta, Georgia. She is a licensed psychologist with eighteen years of clinical experience and is currently the Assistant Director of the Employee Assistance Program at Emory University. She has published over a dozen articles in academic journals and other university publications.